WHAT THE PROS ARE S̶ THINK SAFE

"Jim has written a comprehensive, well-researched crime prevention manual that is as valuable to the protection professional as it is to the average citizen."

— Chief Jeff Wesley
Denham Springs Police Department
Denham Springs, Louisiana

"The statistics are frightening, but the advice is solid. This is the resource you need to be safe in uncertain times."

— Mark Stivers, Captain
Sunnyvale Department of Public Safety
Sunnyvale, California

"Jim McGrew's book is important reading for anyone whose parents or elder loved ones may require long-term or skilled nursing homecare. Armed with this information and contemporary material about individual facilities available from public sources, watch dog groups, and state agencies, family members can make more informed decisions about their care choices."

— Elliot Boxerbaum, CPP, President
Security/Risk Management Consultants, Inc.

"As a women's jail commander, I have had contact with hundreds of victims of domestic violence which led to a downward spiral in their life. I wish they could have had the information in Jim's book which could have prevented that result."

— T.K. Davis, Deputy Chief of Operations (retired)
Santa Clara County Department of Corrections, California

"Jim's experience in law enforcement and security makes *Think Safe* a valuable and practical guide to personal and workplace safety and security."

— Broadus Durant (retired)
Hospital Security and Transportation Manager

"Every organization, large or small, can benefit from Jim's sound advice. Awareness is one of the best methods for preventing workplace violence and harassment before it starts, and Jim provides a practical framework that can work in any environment. I thought Jim made an excellent point about workplace violence with regard to statistics and cases that make national headlines: for the majority of employers, these 'sensational' types of events are not what they will encounter. Very often, the behavior will be subtle, and may take years to surface. Jim gives practical advice on behavioral cues and traits, along with situations that might be okay to handle and where to ask for assistance."

— Nancy C. Nelson
Human Resources Director
Ultra Clean Technology

"No matter where we live, we are all subject to personal safety and security risks – whether at our places of work, while in public, or even while in our own homes. *Think Safe* outlines many of the risks and describes scenarios that serve to increase our awareness. But more importantly, *Think Safe* offers us practical advice on taking effective countermeasures. Thanks Jim, for sharing your extensive experience and superior professional know-how."

— Rick Daniels, MA (criminology), CPP, CFE
International Security Consultant

Think
Safe

Practical Measures to Increase
Security at Home, at Work,
and Throughout Life.

James M. McGrew, CPP, CFE

04 05 06 HH 10 9 8 7 6 5 4 3 1
First Edition
Printed in the United States of America
ISBN-10: 0-9744149-6-4
ISBN-13: 978-0-9744149-6-4
$19.95-US
Library of Congress Control #: 2004116010

Requests for permission to make copies of any part of this work can be made to:

Cameo Publications, LLC.
PO Box 8006
Hilton Head Island, SC 29938
1-866-372-2636
info@cameopublications.com
www.cameopublications.com

Edited by Melinda Copp of Cameo Publications.
The cover and interior text were designed by
David Josephson, CTM, of Cameo Publications.

To Judy, my wonderful wife, friend, and best fishing buddy.

About the Author

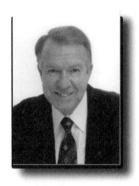

As president and CEO of a full-service investigative and security consulting firm in San Jose, California, James McGrew has over thirty years of experience in planning, implementing, and managing security programs in both the public and private sectors.

As a law enforcement officer, Jim investigated crimes against children, women, and other sex crimes. As a crime prevention officer, he presented hundreds of lectures on burglary prevention, self protection for women, and fraud prevention.

After serving as a law enforcement officer, Jim worked in management and security for several different companies. He worked his way up through the ranks, and eventually became a high-level manager of a Fortune 500 company.

During his corporate career, Jim developed his ability to evaluate and execute investigative assignments. His techniques are designed to fit the needs and styles of corporate entities, such as human resources, legal departments, and top tier management. Jim has used his experience to develop effective protocols and successfully teamed with other senior level managers to investigate fraud, theft, conflicts of interest, and other ethical violations of domestic and international scope.

Stressing the value and implementation of risk assessment, Jim has applied his expertise to corporate security, high-tech manufacturing, healthcare safety and security, and corporate investigations. His pro-active management programs have successfully addressed violence in the workplace, travel safety, emergency action and contingency plans, and other vital security issues.

Jim is a Certified Protection Professional, a Certified Fraud Examiner, a Private Investigator licensed by the State of California, and he earned his Masters degree in Administration of Justice from San Jose State.

Prey ... (noun) a victim; an animal hunted or caught for food; (verb) to seize as prey; to victimize; to plunder.

Prey in many circumstances is necessary for continued existence. A fox preys on the rabbit for food. Similarly, a bird devours various insects to survive. Human predators are concerned only with themselves, and they act only out of selfishness. The act of preying on a victim satisfies feelings of sexual desire, revenge, anger, and retaliation in predators. No pages of this book are devoted to the causes of these desires in humans to prey; that is for others. This work emphasizes actions and strategies to reduce the likelihood of being targeted as "easy prey."

Thanks to Laurie Larkins. Without her commitment, perseverance, and attention to detail, this work would not have been possible. ·

Thanks to my friends who offered encouragement.

Thanks to Melinda Copp and David Josephson of Cameo Publications for their expert guidance and support along the way.

And thanks to my customers for their confidence and loyalty.

CONTENTS

PREFACE..XVII

SECTION ONE -
SAFETY PRECAUTIONS FOR PARENTS 19

Chapter 1: THE INFANT...25
HOSPITAL PRECAUTIONS 26
PARENTAL PRECAUTIONS 26
OTHER PARENTAL CONSIDERATIONS 27
VISITORS 28

Chapter 2: CHILDCARE 29
OTHER CAREGIVER QUALIFIERS 31
SELECTION IS A LENGTHY PROCESS................................32

Chapter 3: SCHOOL- AGE CHILDREN 37
SCHOOL VIOLENCE 39
NON-FATAL TEACHER VICTIMIZATION..........................41
NATIONAL CENTER FOR EDUCATION STATISTICS 42
WORK PLACE VIOLENT VICTIMIZATION 43
STRATEGIES/ACTIONS FOR PARENTS AND THE OLDER CHILD 44
TEENAGE DEPRESSION 47
SUICIDE INTERVENTION 48

Chapter 4: BABYSITTERS 49
GUIDE FOR PARENTS...49
GUIDE FOR BABYSITTERS 50

Chapter 5: ON-LINE PARENTING 53
MANAGING INTERNET USE 54
STRATEGIES FOR PARENTS 55
WEB SAFETY TIPS FOR CHILDREN 55
WARNING SIGNALS 56

Chapter 6: COLLEGE CONSIDERATIONS 57

Section Two -
Safety Precautions for Women 59
Victimization by age, gender, and Crime 60

Chapter 7: College Considerations -
Especially for Women 61
Date Rape 62
Defenses 62
Rape of College Women 63
Prevention Strategies 63
Stalkers 64
Prevention Strategies 64

Chapter 8: Rape Defense 67
Many Victims Know Their Rapist 67
Attacks in the Home 68
Safety at Home 69
Other precautions 70
Precautions in and around a vehicle 71
Sexual Assaults 71
Rape Trauma 73
Police and Prosecution 73

Chapter 9: Domestic Violence 75
The Cycle of Violence 76
The Batterer 77
Court Process and Legal Terms 77
Recognizing Signs/Symptoms of Domestic Violence 79
Breaking the Cycle of Violence 79

Section Three -
Safety Precautions for the Elderly 81
Chapter 10: Crimes Against the Elderly 83
Elder Abuse 83
Physical Abuse 84
Sexual Abuse 84

PSYCHOLOGICAL ABUSE 84
FINANCIAL (FIDUCIARY) ABUSE 84
ABUSERS OF THE ELDERLY 86
THE VICTIMS 86
CAUSES OF DOMESTIC ELDER ABUSE 86
PREVENTING ELDER ABUSE 87

Chapter 11: FINANCIAL / FIDUCIARY ABUSE 89
COMMON SCAMS AND SCHEMES 90
THE PIGEON DROP 90
BANK EXAMINER FRAUD 90
SWEETHEART SWINDLE 91
HOME REPAIR 91
HIRING A CONTRACTOR 92
TELEMARKETING – HELP IS ON THE WAY................................93
CANADIAN SWEEPSTAKES SCAM 93
PHONY VEHICLE ACCIDENT 94
DISTRACTION BURGLARY 94
MAGAZINE SUBSCRIPTIONS...95
CREDIT AND CHARGE CARD FRAUD/THEFT 97
CAREGIVER THEFT 98
ELDERLY PEOPLE AND INVESTMENT FRAUD 98
PROMISSORY NOTES 98
INTERNET FRAUD 99
TELEMARKETING FRAUD 99
VIATICAL INVESTMENTS.. 100
ENTERTAINMENT SCAMS.. 100
PONZI/PYRAMID SCHEMES 101
AVOID INVESTMENT FRAUD 101
CREDIT CARD FRAUD PREVENTION..103
WARNING SIGNS OF FINANCIAL EXPLOITATION.................. 104

SECTION FOUR -
SAFETY PRECAUTIONS AT WORK 107

Chapter 12: WORKPLACE VIOLENCE.....................109
WARNING SIGNS OF VIOLENT INDIVIDUALS 110
RECOGNIZING INAPPROPRIATE BEHAVIOR 111
HIGH RISK BEHAVIOR TO WATCH FOR 112
STRATEGIES TO DE-ESCALATE POTENTIALLY VIOLENT SITUATIONS.113
THINGS TO DO AND <u>NOT</u> DO 113

Chapter 13: SEXUAL HARASSMENT 115
QUID PRO QUO SEXUAL HARASSMENT 115
HOSTILE ENVIRONMENT SEXUAL HARASSMENT.............................116

SECTION FIVE -
CONSUMER FRAUD PREVENTION...........................119

Chapter 14: CONSUMER FRAUD...........................121
MAGAZINE SUBSCRIPTION SCAMS 121
TELEMARKETING TRAVEL FRAUD..122
BANK DEBIT AND CHARGE CARDS 123
SWEEPSTAKES FRAUD 124
CHARITABLE DONATIONS 125
FRAUDULENT LOAN BROKERS 125
CREDIT CARD PROTECTION SCAM..126
INVESTMENT FRAUD 127
REDUCE EXPOSURE TO FRAUD..128

Chapter 15: IDENTITY THEFT 129
IF YOU ARE A VICTIM OF IDENTITY THEFT....................................131
OTHER STEPS TO TAKE 132

SECTION SIX -
GENERAL SAFETY PRECAUTIONS 133

Chapter 16: WEAPONS FOR DEFENSE 135
SELF DEFENSE CLASSES - PRACTICAL USEFULNESS........................135
CHEMICAL SPRAY...135

Hand Guns 136

Chapter 17: Carjacking 137
High Risk Situations 137
Risk Reduction around Your Car 138
Risk Reduction While Driving 138
Risk Reduction When Parking 138

Chapter 18: Personal Threats 139
Personal Threats at Work 142

Section Seven -
Crime Prevention 145

Chapter 19: Protecting the Home 147
The Relationship between Physical Security Measures
and Security Functions 149
Security Devices and Systems 149
Doors 150
Windows and Sliding Glass Doors 151
Lighting 152
Perimeter and Structural Security 153
Home Security – A Dog 158
Property Identification 159
Burglar Alarms 160
Security Survey 161

Residential Survey 162

Conclusion 164

Index.. 165

Think Safe

Practical Measures to Increase
Security at Home, at Work,
and Throughout Life.

James M. McGrew, CPP, CFE

PREFACE

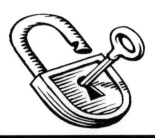

Criminologists, psychologists, sociologists, and a host of others have contributed volumes of scientific study on crime and criminals. And some degree of understanding the causative factors of crime in our society has resulted from these studies. For example, abusive or violent child rearing practices produce a higher likelihood of the child being abusive or violent as an adult. But pragmatically speaking, this information is insignificant to a victim of a violent crime, or the victim's family.

The victims of violent crime and their family members don't care how the criminal who hurt them was raised, especially in cases of murder, rape, and child molestation. Understanding a criminal's upbringing does not repair damage, or bring back a child or loved one. Until society's experts can intervene with care and treatment from a preventative perspective, you must employ other strategies to protect the family, home, and community from those who prey on them. Ideally, these strategies should be developed from scientific study, be practical in application, and reduce the chance of becoming a victim.

This book will offer some basic safety strategies that everyone should use to keep their families, homes, and themselves safe from predators. In addition, real-life experiences utilized throughout this book add value and perspective on contemporary crime issues, and mitigate risk.

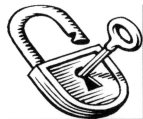

Section One –
Safety Precautions
for Parents

- CHAPTER 1 - THE INFANT
- CHAPTER 2 - CHILDCARE
- CHAPTER 3 - SCHOOL-AGE CHILDREN INTERVENTION
- CHAPTER 4 - BABYSITTERS
- CHAPTER 5 - ON-LINE PARENTING
- CHAPTER 6 - COLLEGE CONSIDERATIONS

Introduction

Personal safety is extremely important for parents. Because beyond caring for themselves, parents are also responsible for the safety and well-being of their children. Unfortunately, many parents don't emphasize safety enough, until it's too late. Every night, the news broadcasts stories of missing children, child abuse, break-ins, and violence in schools. When parents don't teach their children how to be safe in different situations, the results may be tragic.

The following Bureau of Justice Violent Crime Statistics concerning victims of murder, rape, and assault illustrates that, in general, the younger the person, the more likely they are to experience a violent crime. Persons age

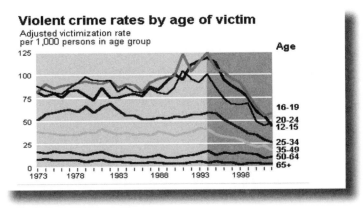

Figure 1

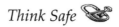

All crimes against children are unconscionable. But sexual assault against children is perhaps the most feared in our society. **The National Incident-Based Reporting System** (NIBRS) regarding sexual assault reports (Table 1):

☐ Sixty-seven percent of all victims of sexual assault reported to law enforcement agencies were juveniles (under the age of eighteen).

☐ One of every seven victims of sexual assaults (or fourteen percent of all victims) reported to law enforcement agencies were under age six.

☐ Forty percent of the offenders who victimized children under the age of six were juveniles themselves.

Table 1. Age profile of the victims of sexual assault

Victim age	All sexual assault	Forcible rape	Forcible sodomy	Sexual assault with object	Forcible fondling
Total	100.0%	100.0%	100.0%	100.0%	100.0%
0 to 5	14.0%	4.3%	24.0%	26.5%	20.2%
6 to 11	20.1	8.0	30.8	23.2	29.3
12 to 17	32.8	33.5	24.0	25.5	34.3
18 to 24	14.2	22.6	8.7	9.7	7.7
25 to 34	11.5	19.6	7.5	8.3	5.0
Above 34	7.4	12.0	5.1	6.8	3.5

Section 1 - Introduction

☐ Thirty-four percent of all victims of sexual assault were under age twelve (Figure 2).

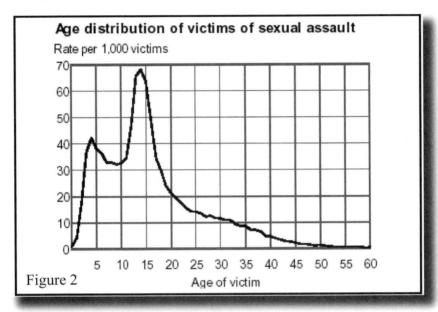

Age distribution of victims of sexual assault

Rate per 1,000 victims

Figure 2 — Age of victim

☐ Females in the NIBRS Report were more than six times (or eighty-six percent) as likely as males to be victims of sexual assaults (Figure 3).

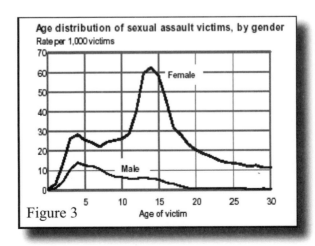

Age distribution of sexual assault victims, by gender

Rate per 1,000 victims

Figure 3 — Age of victim

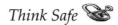

☐ For victims under age twelve, males were assaulted with an object nineteen percent, forcible fondling twenty-six percent, and forcible sodomy sixty-four percent. Based on these findings, males are most likely to be a victim of a sexual assault at age four (Figure 4). As a male's age increases, victimization decreases.

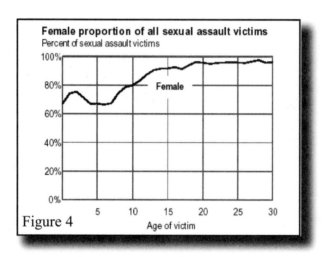

Figure 4

Section 1 - Introduction

☐ Sexual assaults are categorized into four areas: forcible rape, forcible sodomy, sexual assault with an object, and forcible fondling. Age profiles for these assaults are found in Figure 5.

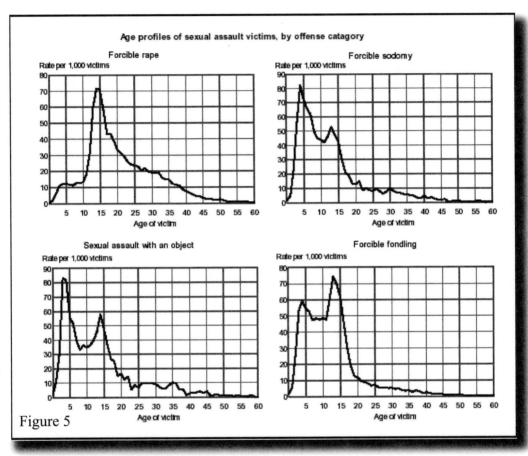

Figure 5

The above information comes from a NIBRS Statistical Report – Sexual Assault of Young Children as Reported to Law Enforcement: Victim, Incident, and Offender Characteristics by Howard N. Snyder, PH.D., National Center for Juvenile Justice, July 2000, NCJ 182990.

These statistics are nothing less than frightening, and they only support the need for solid safety precautions where children are concerned. The first section of this book is devoted to the safety precautions parents should use to ensure the safety of their families. Each chapter covers a different stage of the child's life, and explains what parents should expect from their children when they reach that stage. When parents use the safety precautions contained in each chapter, they greatly reduce the risk for their children to become victims of crime.

Chapter 1

THE INFANT

Your parental role begins shortly after conception and well before birth—near conception by spreading the wonderful news, remodeling the home, shopping for baby clothes, physical body changes, and all the actions you take and behavioral patterns that change when planning for a new baby. And each of these changes can clue-in potential abductors. Often during this pre-birth period, the abductor preys on the excitement and subsequent lower defense mechanisms of the expectant mother to establish acquaintance. After all, how many expectant mothers would not engage in conversation about their blessed event?

A potential abductor with average skill can collect an enormous amount of personal information if the respondent is unaware. Information such as doctor's name and address, due date, perhaps the baby's gender, delivery hospital, number and ages of other children in the family, stay-at-home parent or childcare, address of childcare facility, and more.

Other vulnerable areas include birth announcements in local newspapers or work bulletin boards that contain personal information such as addresses or pictures. Be cautious of free offers either by mail or telephone. Abductors may use these offers as bait to get private information on your family. Tactics the infant abductor may utilize are watching the hospitals and doctors offices, checking birth announcements, posing as hospital employees, caregivers, etc.

Potentially harmful social interactions occur all the time, everyday in supermarket checkouts, clothing stores, theatre lines, etc. People see an expectant mother and want to know when she's expecting, or whether it's a boy or a girl. A friendly inquiry in a public setting may seem harmless, and is usually without significance. But those interactions with significance can have terrible consequences. You never really know why a stranger wants to know about your pregnancy. They may just want to congratulate you, or maybe they're just curious, but you can never be sure.

Control and limit the information (intelligence) you give to strangers in such situations. Respond to questions, but leave out the specifics. Don't tell anyone where the baby will be delivered, or by which doctor, and especially not where you live. This practice is incredibly important because over one third of infant abductions occur in the home.

Hospital Precautions

Protecting your infant against abduction, or infant prey, requires a collaboration of parents and healthcare providers in hospitals. Healthcare providers are the forefront of safety and security for the infant and mother. And security in the hospital environment poses a major challenge for staff, due to the nature of activity within the perimeter of most newborn units, i.e., new parents, their relatives, visitors, students, volunteers, among others. They create an ever-changing facial landscape in an open, high traffic environment.

Consequently, recognizing a potential abductor is problematic because he/she can easily simulate a role consistent with the hospital environment, like a new nurse, or visiting family member. Often a feigned role provides the cover for the abductor to gain access to mother and child. However, several strategies are effective in mitigating risk to the newborn and mother, such as a comprehensive plan of action for each healthcare group that comes in contact with a newborn. Additionally, each part of the plan must synchronize efforts to deter or detect abduction.

One method of deterrence is employee identification badges. Badges should be specific to those in contact with newborns and sufficiently distinguishable for mothers to recognize as authorized infant care personnel. Similarly, temporary badges for permitted visitors or volunteers around infants help to distinguish their role, relationship, and authority. Become familiar with the hospital staff name badges, so you can easily spot any inconsistencies or fakes.

While name badges may be the primary method of deterrence, some hospitals also take extra precautions such as discontinuing birth announcements in newspapers, conducting periodic security reviews of protection measures, and regularly testing those measures to insure they work.

Parental Precautions

Parental participation in preventing hospital abductions is critical to complete the circle of protection for the infant. The most opportune time to discuss safety protocol with the hospital staff is before delivery. This may be accomplished by requesting written guidelines, or aspects of the hospital security plan that affect the parent and/or the newborn. These written guidelines then become Items of Action between the hospital and parent. Expect to see *Items of Action* similar to the following:

- ☐ Review and understand the hospital infant security plan.

- ☐ Always keep the infant within parental view.

- ☐ Always keep the infant opposite the entrance door.

- ☐ Never give the infant to anyone without an appropriate badge.

- ☐ Challenge unfamiliar persons inquiring about your infant.

- ☐ Accompany the infant if medical needs require relocation.

- ☐ Take a color photograph and record a full description of the infant.

- ☐ Fingerprint and apply a bracelet/anklet to the infant.

Other Parental Considerations

Carefully weigh risk factors before publicly announcing your child's birth. Those that prey on a child (or home) read birth, death, and social announcements. If you do decide to publicly announce the birth of your baby, provide minimum information, such as, "The Jones of Smithtown, NJ, are proud to welcome the new addition to their family." Similarly, banners on lawns, garages, etc. could provide an opportunity for serious trouble. The main idea is to attract a minimum amount of attention, despite your excitement and desire to share your joy with the world.

The best defense for the infant in the home is to keep out potential abductors. Often home and personal safety/security is not a high priority prior to arrival of an infant. But after you bring your baby home, it should be your main concern. Thus a review of your existing security systems is probably in order.

At minimum, all existing door and window locks should be in working order. Emergency phone numbers should be posted near phones. Fire extinguishers should be checked for degree of charge, or purchased if none exist in the dwelling. Smoke detectors should be checked, and a light timer utilized, if available. Additional home security measures are covered in section seven.

Visitors

Visitors fall in three categories: unauthorized, authorized friendly, and authorized unfriendly. Unauthorized are kept out with locks, alarms, and other security devices. Authorized friendly visitors are non-threatening and may include family members, relatives, close friends, or clergy. Authorized unfriendly visitors pose a particular threat because the person has disguised his/her intent with a legitimate cover. Examples of legitimate cover could be anything associated with a complete or partial uniform, such as a nurse, mailperson, or delivery person.

Additionally, these unauthorized unfriendly visitors often use a ruse of a personal emergency to gain entrance, such as a lost dog, flat tire, need of telephone, etc. Use extreme caution in these circumstances, because once inside your dwelling, the intruder may create a distraction to divert your attention and abduct an infant. This diversion need only last a minute or two because these attacks are carefully pre-planned for execution. Do not allow unauthorized or unfriendly people entry into the dwelling. Accommodate their request for assistance in another way.

Chapter 2

CHILDCARE

Millions of children in the United States participate in activities provided by public and private organizations each year, such as public nonprofit or private daycare, home daycare, and structured or non-structured care. Your selection of service is an individual choice based on several factors, price being an important issue. However, as you select your childcare service, you should always consider whether the environment is safe, secure, and healthy for your child.

States regulate childcare providers in a number of ways. Licensing or registration is a primary function. And the state's records are relatively easy to access by telephone or Internet. Always check to make sure a service is appropriately licensed or registered.

Criminal history record checks are one of several methods used to predict the suitability of individuals seeking paid or volunteer positions that interact with children. National fingerprint checks can show the criminal history of any individual convicted of a crime anywhere in the United States, who seeks a volunteer or paid position in any state.

A law enacted in 1993, **The National Child Protection Act**, authorizes the FBI to exchange identification records with state and local officials for licensing and employment purposes, provided exchanges are also authorized by a state statute that has been approved by the U.S. Attorney General. Thus any state that wants the FBI to conduct national criminal history checks of childcare or youth service workers must have a law defining what categories of jobs or positions require background checks and these background checks must be based on fingerprints.

National fingerprint-based checks are not quantifiable; but the deterrent effect of a national criminal background check utilizing fingerprints is logically significant. So as soon as a person finds out the position requires a background check, they don't apply for it. Experience in drug testing seems similar in nature, and often an applicant once advised of the drug screen requirement, never shows up again. Obviously, other factors may account for a no-show, but reasonably not all cases are coincidental. All considered, the deterrent effect of national background checks keeps unsuitable applicants from childcare related positions.

Several other considerations in the screening process are equally important to the applicant's background, e.g. previous work history, references, and local and state records, particularly driver's records if transportation is applicable. Additionally, a driver's record may detect aggressive behavior, such as reckless driving, driving while intoxicated, or perhaps even road rage issues. But keep in mind, the record is only as good as the accuracy of the input. If a record is incomplete, or an error occurred in documentation, it may not be reliable.

Fundamentally, national fingerprint-based background checks may be the only effective way to identify the worst abusers of children. Pedophiles that move from state to state, change names, and conceal identities can be exposed through fingerprint checks. Similarly, national checks can identify criminal histories involving other offenses that may affect a person's reliability in working with children, such as drug possession or sales, assault/battery, acts of violence, or theft.

Examples of value with national fingerprint-based checks are numerous:

☐ A national background check discovered an applicant for a special education teaching position had been convicted of rape in another state.

☐ A national fingerprint check of non-instructional staff resulted in several terminations. Each had record(s) of a serious offense inappropriate to interaction with children.

☐ Fingerprint searches of potential foster parents over a period of time, identified over nine percent with felony records.

Background checks must be an integral piece of the qualifications inquiry for childcare providers and/or any person who interacts with children in a care-oriented environment.

In 2002, California's Governor Gray Davis sponsored emergency regulations giving parents the right to know whether childcare providers have criminal records. Previously, people with serious criminal behavior, such as drug dealing and indecent exposure, could obtain childcare licensing. Additionally, "exceptions" for certain criminal acts, such as shoplifting and non-felony convictions, were unavailable and confidential. These emergency rules were implemented to give parents the right to obtain the names of childcare workers "with exceptions" and to reduce the possibility of felons obtaining childcare licensing.

To publicize and promote the regulations, the law requires childcare providers to notify the parents who must sign off the notification of their rights. As currently written, parents can't learn the specific crimes that exist in the records. However, legal efforts to grant parents access to a careworker's specific criminal violations continue.

Other Caregiver Qualifiers

Expect to find varying levels of quality from childcare facility to childcare facility. These levels of quality seem to relate to comparable factors, such as:

- ☐ **The number of children to number of staff.** The better the ratio of staff to children means the greater the likelihood of appropriate care in addition to health and safety.

- ☐ **Written procedures establishing core care for all children.** These procedures should become a business model for all care-givers to adhere. The model may include items such as disciplinary procedures for severe and/or inappropriate misconduct, reporting of injury or suspicious marks on the child's body, and how to deal with suspected abuse or neglect.

- ☐ **Positive attitudes.** Pleasant environments mean more than toys and games to play for the child. And a positive attitude of the staff tends to result in positive behavior from the child. Probably every-one can recall people in their lives who made a considerable impact on their childhood through a positive attitude toward people and things, and you naturally want the same positive experiences for your children. Part of childcare staff evaluations should include an element considering attitudinal factors. A parent may get a good feeling for the general attitude held in a facility by visiting it (both announced and unannounced) and watching the interactions between staff members and children.

- ☐ **Staff training.** Training should minimally encompass discipline and misbehavior strategies, behavior modification, and preven-

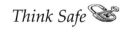

tion of child abuse and sexual molestation. Training should be documented and recorded in personnel folders.

☐ **Evaluation and audit.** Each childcare facility should have a system for monitoring staff-child ratios, compliance to policies and procedures, and employee attitudes and performance. Annual internal audits are invaluable in tracking performance with objectives, and for developing strategies for improvement as required.

Obviously, you want to find the best available care for your child or children within your financial means. So consider each of these factors when making your decision.

Selection is a Lengthy Process

A place to begin the search for the best available service is through referral. Ask your friends and co-workers where they take their children, or if they have any suggestions or insights. Develop a list of referrals that seem to approximate your needs. Besides geography and cost, other factors, such as matching job hours with hours of service, may affect the list.

Second, develop a series of preliminary questions that fill the needs in your individual childcare situation. These questions will serve as pre-qualifiers to manage the referral list down to a preferred list. A spreadsheet may be developed with the preferred facility in one column and responses to questions in another set of columns. A computer simplifies this task; however pencil and paper work just fine. Some questions that may appear on the list are:

☐ Is there a waiting list? If so, how long?

☐ How many children are currently under care?

☐ What is the ratio of staff to child?

☐ Are you insured? Verify with the insuring agency.

☐ Are staff and support personnel background checked? To what degree?

☐ Are there written Policies and Procedures?

☐ Is there a disciplinary process for employees?

☐ What is the experience level of each caregiver?

Chapter 2 - Childcare

☐ What precautions are taken to reduce risk of child abuse?

☐ Do you allow unannounced visits by parents?

☐ What is the disciplinary process for children?

☐ Are children taken on day trips? If so, who provides care? Transportation?

Children require the protection of adults, but often times they also require protection from adults. Review the questions above, and understand why they are critical to the pre-qualification investigation. The answers provided by the caregiver, and also the manner in which they were given, should establish a preferred list for further consideration. Most importantly, you should evaluate the answers to your questions, and feel confident that they meet your expectations before investigating a childcare facility any further.

Next, arrange a visit to the childcare facility for an inspection. Begin your inspection from the outside. Drive around the facility, maybe around a block or two. Notice the condition of the surrounding neighborhood and the outside condition of the childcare facility. Are lawns cared for, buildings painted, and fences in good condition? Also, notice the condition of playground equipment. You should visually check fastening devices for swings, slides, and other pieces of climbing equipment. Also, look to see if any play equipment is "out of order." Through observation, you should get a general feeling about the condition of the facility. Additionally, look for attractive nuisances such as lawn tools, lawn mowers, and similar dangerous devices that may attract youngsters.

Once inside, look at the floor surface and the general cleanliness of the facility. Check for safety equipment, First-Aid kits, fire extinguishers, fire sprinklers, and safety procedures such as evacuation plans. Determine if written emergency plans exist, and if they are reviewed as part of an annual audit. Are plans practiced and updated? Ask how many First-Aid/CPR trained staff members are available. At least one staff person should be fully certified.

Communicable diseases at daycare centers are a serious concern for staff and child. A policy concerning personal hygiene, from basic hand washing to immunizations, can reduce illness in the childcare setting. Healthcare nurses often work with daycare staff to establish effective illness prevention programs with guidelines and methods to reduce infections. As a parent, you should inquire about illness prevention programs in each childcare facility you visit.

Evaluate staff relationships to each other for politeness, courtesy, respect, and other mannerisms that children learn from example. Ask to see written Policies and Procedures. Inquire about staff disciplinary actions related to violation of policy or procedure. Ask for an example of a recent action. Look for examples that take on a positive approach of corrective action/s. Ask yourself if it were you involved, would you likely receive the corrective action as part of a learning process, or view it as entirely disciplinary in nature. Ideally, the corrective action/s should be constructive in nature and encourage the staff person to strive for personal satisfaction in doing a better job.

Ask about staff turnover. Frequent turnover may be related to unpleasant working conditions and unhappy employees. Also, turnover rates provide a baseline for future checks on employee relations. If the turnover suddenly shifts higher, something may be wrong internally.

Listen to the words of your escort, but also watch the children. Do they seem happy or tentative, reserved or gregarious? Their actions will give a sense of what their life at the facility is really like.

Do not hesitate to ask about child abuse prevention and detection. Unfortunately, no environment is completely immune. People who prey on children are in childcare, churches, schools, organized sports, service clubs, and elsewhere.

Policies that aid in prevention are: 1) personnel selection process, e.g. fingerprint background checks, reference checks given by candidates and references developed independently and if possible, verification of degrees; 2) education of children at the earliest age concerning their body; and 3) an open opportunity for dialogue about child abuse, its early recognition and intervention within an organization.

Policies that aid in detection are: 1) inspect the children daily; 2) notation of bruises, injuries, or sensitivity to touch; and 3) a system for reacting accordingly to abuse indications, including getting an explanation from a responsible person about how the bruise or injury occurred, and reporting unexplained or suspicious circumstances to the local police authorities.

As you move through the selection process, you should begin to get a feel for the facility and develop additional questions such as, how well are programs suited to your child's learning. And is the program content consistent with what you want your child to learn?

After you have chosen the facility that best fits your needs, the job is not complete. In some respects, this is just the beginning.

The safety and security of your child depends on two things: One, your investigation to select the best possible provider in your circumstances, and two, regular follow-ups, unannounced visits to see the child's real world situation, physical inspection of the child, and as appropriate, talking with the child about his/her daily experiences.

Chapter 2 - Childcare

Parents must remember they cannot abdicate responsibility for their child to the childcare center in totality. Center personnel will turnover, things will change, and problems will arise. You should visit the center as often as possible with a critical eye toward evaluating the environment. If possible, parents should alter the time of day of a visit in order to get a complete picture of the children's activities.

Should something be of concern, act immediately and discuss the issue with the center management. Also, you should establish a follow-up date for notification that your concern has been addressed. Shortly thereafter, revisit the facility and verify for yourself that the issue has been resolved to your satisfaction. Obviously, if a concern is dangerous to the child, remove the child immediately.

Chapter 3   SCHOOL-AGE CHILDREN

T wo bills introduced in the 107th Congress, the **HR 1812 School Anti-Violence Empowerment Act** and the **HR 1216 Comprehensive School Safety Act**, represent both the continuing danger to school children and efforts to reduce that danger. Bill **HR 1812** provides grants for local educational agencies to establish or enhance intervention programs and school safety programs for students, staff, and school facilities. Priorities for ward grants are based on existing or proposed violence prevention programs and crisis intervention counseling services, among other administrative services. It also allocates 750 million dollars for cooperative partnerships between schools and state and local police departments to provide police officers in schools.

Bill **HR 1216** also provides for grants to state educational agencies to implement school safety plans. A local agency may apply for a sub-grant for funds, but it limits administrative costs to not more than 1.5 percent. Funds are to be used for three purposes:

1) Assess current school crime committed on school campuses and school-related functions;

2) Identify strategies and programs for a high level of school safety;

3) Provide a safe and orderly environment conducive to learning. These bills represent the government recognition of the need to continue efforts toward developing programs, services, and strategies for addressing crime on the school grounds.

As discussed earlier, protection strategies begin with infancy and continue as the parental responsibility to nurture the basic awareness of personal protection in their child, prior to beginning school. Some examples may be obvious such as learning their full name and address, the rules of telephone usage, their

37

private body parts and what to do if they are touched inappropriately, how to deal with strangers, and how to look both ways when crossing streets. These protective measures prepare your child for periods of time when they are absent adult supervision, such as walking to and from school.

The *San Jose Mercury News* ran a story on Wednesday, September 4, 2002 about a young girl accosted on the way to school by two men in a van.

"These things occur periodically," said the school principal in the article, "but it seems they're on the increase, and when it happens in your own community you realize it can happen anywhere."

The girl reported a passenger in the van demanded she get in, but instead she ran toward her school. She thought she was safe until the van reappeared and the passenger repeated the demand. The little girl remembered her mom's advice, "always run," and she ran inside the school. In this instance, mom and daughter agreed to a plan of action and the daughter executed it successfully. If they hadn't formulated this plan, and if the mother didn't reiterate the importance of running from strangers to her daughter, this story may have ended in tragedy.

This plan worked for this family and perhaps will work for others. When devising a plan for your family members, remember that it doesn't have to be complicated. Effective plans can be as simple as walking against traffic. This action alone forces a vehicle to go on the wrong side of the road to attempt abduction by force. Parents may also help children by identifying safe houses for refuge. Fire stations and police stations are ideal safe locations. Other safe houses may include neighborhood watch homes, which are generally identified with signage. Also, parents can work with school officials to arrange for a police crime prevention officer to visit the school and discuss crimes against children. Cell phones with emergency numbers pre-programmed can also be an effective tool for older children.

But the key factor in the safe progression of a child through the school years is to start early. Talk to your children about taking shortcuts to school, accepting rides from people without your approval, and how to decline an offer for anything contrary to your agreement. Practicing your plan is critically important because predators rely on the child's inexperience to develop scenarios that prompt the child to make a bad decision. Examples of scenarios could be: "Your parent(s) have been injured. You must come with me," or "Your teacher wants you back at school, come with me."

Another ploy is pets. Small kittens may be used to entice youngsters into dangerous situations. Discuss these kinds of situations with your children often enough for them to understand that adults may try to trick them into going with them. Provide them with alternatives. Most important, whatever alternative you agree upon, test it to insure it works. It's also a good idea to have a back up to your alternative, maybe a second option for a safe house or some other outlet for your child to find safety.

Whatever you and your child decide, make sure you keep the plan as simple as possible. Complex plans seldom work in an emergency. And if your children forget or ignore your agreement or plan, correct the behavior by explaining how much you love and care for them, and how you worry during their unexplained absence. Repeat your plan with them regularly, because investing time to stress personal safety with children at every stage of development pays dividends. Most important, no substitute for parental guidance exists in a child's life, so parents must be involved.

School Violence

Children of all ages are harmed in many ways. Internet access to sexually-oriented sites, drug promotion, and bomb making are clearly a concern; however, other dangers abound:

The following was excerpted from the *Contra Costa Times* in Northern California on September 24, 2002:

> Police are looking for a man suspected of assaulting and sexually molesting a 14-year-old student he abducted from a parking lot at a local middle school before the start of morning school.

> On August 31, 2004, the *San Jose Mercury News* reported a plea agreement for a drug dealer who gave the drug Ecstasy to a seventeen-year-old girl who in turn gave it to three middle school girls. One of the three girls experimented with the drug while at a slumber party, overdosed and died. The two other girls watched the event and didn't intervene. Medical personnel say she would have survived if help had been called.

Children are exposed to criminal threats to their personal safety like these examples in class, at school-related functions, and on their way to and from school. Violence in U.S. schools mirrors violence in society and almost every crime committed in our society has also been committed on a school ground. Government studies of violent deaths at school, non-fatal student victimization, theft, and crime in school, police reports, and non-fatal teacher victimization at school provide insight into the problems and possible strategies for child protection.

In study year 1997, there were fifty-eight school-associated violent deaths in the United States. Victimization of children ages twelve to eighteen was generally higher at school, particularly related to theft and non-fatal crime at a rate of 101 crimes per 1,000 students. Over seven percent of students reported being threatened or injured with a weapon, gun, knife, or club at school. Almost fifteen percent of students reported participating in physical fights on school property. Bullying of students occurred at a rate of about ten percent in grades six and seven, five percent in grades eight and nine, and two percent in grades ten through twelve, according to the CDC- National Center for Injury Prevention and Control Abstract (School-Associated Violent Deaths in the US 1994-1999).

These statistics often increase in one area and decrease in another. Tragic situations such as the Columbine School shooting also significantly affect the numbers. As an example, *USA Today* (June 2004) reported forty-eight school deaths in the past school year absent a Columbine-like event. For school years July 1999-June 2000, there were thirty-two school-associated violent deaths, according to the US Department of Education's National Center for Education Statistics Violence and Crime at School – Public School Reports. In other crimes, such as suicides, threats of violence, and attacks on teachers, no significant increases seem to exist.

During the period 1997-2001, teachers also experienced violence in the educational setting. Comparing male versus female teachers, male teachers were more likely to be victims of violent crime. For more statistics on crime in schools appear in detail figures, please refer to the chart on facing page.

Non-Fatal Teacher Victimization

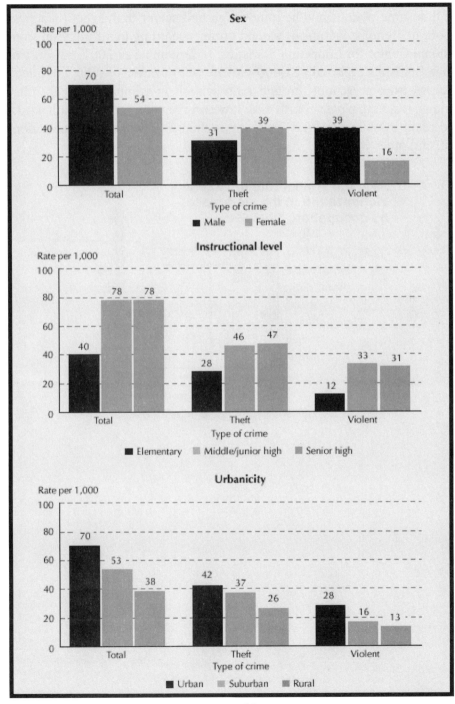

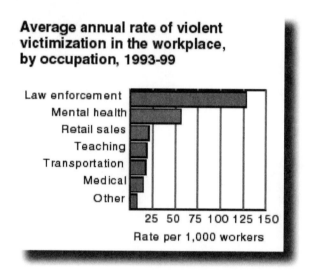

National Center for Education Statistics (NCES)

During this same period, middle/junior high and senior high school teachers were more likely to be victims of violent crime, according to information from the National Center for Education Statistics. In December of 2001, the Bureau of Justice Statistics reported 931,400 violent victimizations in the workplace for teachers from preschool through high school. In comparison with other professions, teaching places fourth after law enforcement, mental health workers, and retail sales in violence. Teaching is then followed by transportation, medical, and other workers.

Average annual rate of violent victimization in the workplace, by occupation, 1993-99

Law enforcement
Mental health
Retail sales
Teaching
Transportation
Medical
Other

25 50 75 100 125 150

Rate per 1,000 workers

Work Place Violent Victimization

Occupational field of victim	Violent victimizations in the workplace		
	Number	Rate per 1,000 workers	Percent of total
Total	12,328,000	12.6	100%
Medical			
Physician	71,300	16.2	0.6%
Nurse	429,100	21.9	3.5
Technician	97,600	12.7	0.8
Other	315,000	8.5	2.6
Mental health			
Professional	290,900	68.2	2.4%
Custodial	60,400	69.0	0.5
Other	186,700	40.7	1.5
Teaching			
Preschool	32,900	7.1	0.3%
Elementary	262,700	16.8	2.1
Junior high	321,300	54.2	2.6
High school	314,500	38.1	2.6
College/university	41,600	1.6	0.3
Technical/industrial	7,400	12.2*	0.1*
Special education	102,000	68.4	0.8
Other	169,800	16.7	1.4
Law enforcement			
Police	1,380,400	260.8	11.2%
Corrections	277,100	155.7	2.3
Private security	369,300	86.6	3.0
Other	359,800	48.3	2.9
Retail sales			
Convenience store	336,800	53.9	2.7%
Gas station	86,900	68.3	0.7
Bartender	170,600	81.6	1.4
Other	1,383,100	15.3	11.2
Transportation			
Bus driver	105,800	38.2	0.9%
Taxi cab driver	84,400	128.3	0.7
Other	350,500	11.7	2.8
Other	4,720,100	7.0	38.3%

Schools should provide an environment of safety and security for students and teachers — one that allows optimum learning and absent of distractions caused by concern for personal safety and/or violent behavior. In real life however, students and teachers are victims of crime and violence at school. Efforts on several fronts to increase safety of teachers and students are underway. But until improvements occur, parents, teachers, and students must increase their own awareness, and develop actions and strategies to deal with this violent reality.

43

Strategies/Actions for Parents and the Older Child

Encourage your children to discuss their daily experiences. These discussions can reveal friends, associates, teachers' names, etc. Always conclude the conversation by asking if there was anything else that happened. Uncovering information about fights, bullying, and other violent behaviors may occur at this point.

Also encourage your children to participate in student projects that promote appropriate, drug-free behavior, such as sports, school programs, and academic clubs. These activities foster healthy, supervised behaviors that will keep your children safe, and will follow them later in life.

One example comes from a November 2002 US Department of Education Report from the Office of Safe and Drug-Free Schools, entitled Student-led Crime Prevention. The student-led crime prevention concept is simple: Young people given the opportunity to take the lead in making their schools safer will benefit both the school and themselves. They also strengthen the school and the school bonds that are essential to their healthy growth as members of the larger community. Student –led crime prevention provides a vehicle to actively engage young people in the life of the school community, to ask for their help and guidance and to offer them the same. It allows those close to the crime problem a means of preventive action.

The program lists the following ten strategies and/or examples of activities for students involved in the program.

1) Report crime and help to make crime reporting a school norm (establish a school reporting system).

2) Help other students with problems (set up a hotline, develop a peer counseling program).

3) Keep the campus physically safe (establish youth patrols or identify problem areas that need attention to the administration).

4) Incorporate crime prevention into existing school clubs or activities (place in such organizations as student council, drama club, art club).

5) Set consequences for violation of school rules or laws (establish a teen court, work to give students a voice in codes of conduct and disciplinary procedures).

6) Help resolve conflict fairly and without violence (establish peer mediation programs and provide conflict mediation/resolution training for all students).

7) Unify the student body by respecting differences and working together (hold town meetings to ensure that everyone's voice is heard, survey students to ensure their concerns are being met).

8) Educate peers and younger youths about preventing issues (establish a cross-age teaching program, encourage the use of cross-age teaching through existing school institutions, and develop education programs for peers).

9) Partner with adults to conduct projects (provide presentations)

10) Use problem-solving teams (respond to specific programs, e.g., vandalism in the locker room, tension among student groups).

The Student-led Crime Prevention Brochure is quite detailed and offers suggestions for implementation, putting principles into action, its benefits, and resource lists, among other valuable information. For a copy of the brochure, fax a request to **1.301.470.1244** or email a request to edpubs@inet.ed.gov.

Another important safety measure for parents is to acknowledge the existence of violent behavior, and discuss factors that contribute to these activities with their children. Parents and students can use the following list to help increase awareness about school violence and the causes:

☐ *Parents:* Discuss how to recognize violent warning signs in others, such as frequent loss of temper, history of fighting, or hurting animals.

☐ *Parents:* Avoid places, things and events that enhance the possibility of risk.

☐ *Parents:* Demand security for after-school functions.

☐ *Parents:* Become a member of, or form a neighborhood watch.

☐ *Parents:* Discuss symptoms of anger and how to keep anger under control and non-violent. Teach your children skills of negotiation and mediation.

Think Safe

☐ *Parents:* Establish expectations of your children for homework, social activities, and other desired behaviors.

☐ *Parents:* Encourage a closed campus policy.

☐ *Parents:* Encourage drug sweeps of the school.

☐ *Parents:* Encourage stationary law enforcement on school property.

☐ *Parents:* Encourage schools to have a formal violence prevention program.

☐ *Parents:* Demand zero tolerance for weapons, gangs, use of alcohol and drugs at school.

☐ *Parents:* Encourage school to provide activities for students during after-school hours and early evening.

☐ *Students:* Report bullies, gang activity, or weapon possession to school authorities.

☐ *Students:* Follow school rules.

☐ *Students:* Travel to and from school with others.

☐ *Students:* Notify parents if you must change a pre-arranged schedule.

☐ *Students:* Students should be encouraged to tell an adult if they see violent warning signs in others.

These actions may require reaching out to School Boards, school administrators, local and state lawmakers, law enforcement, business leaders, national organizations, and district attorneys. Encourage your local politicians and community leaders to start after-school programs that provide sports, tutoring, and educational enrichment for children. Studies by the FBI and youth advocacy groups indicate that as many as fifteen million children have no place to go after school (www.afterschool.gov). Fortunately, a heightened sensitivity to school crime and safety is making a significant contribution in improving data collection. As more data is made available, better and more comprehensive programs for intervention should develop.

Teenage Depression

Perhaps the most challenging parental issue is balancing the demands of society and needs of your family. Many parents are so involved with work and other activities that they have little time left over to deal with issues, other than to feed and clothe family members. But busy or distracted parents neglect family mental health issues. Attention is particularly important during a child's teen-age years in order to identify behaviors that may indicate a number of mental health issues including depression. Consider the following trends in teenage depression:

- ☐ Teens are reporting more serious and complex mental illnesses.

- ☐ Stress and anxiety complaints have replaced less serious complaints with teens.

- ☐ Suicide is the third leading cause of death among fifteen to twenty-four year olds.

Teens and Depression

Recent studies indicate a large number of American teens suffer from depression. ***The Ohio State University Extension Fact Sheet*** Article HYG-5282-95 on Teenage Depression, written by Christine B. Taylor, describes that the difference between "normal" adolescent sadness and clinical depression is based on the time, degree, and amount of deviation from the youth's usual personality and behavior. It seems that absent regular interaction with the teen, it would be very difficult, if not impossible to recognize what is deviant from their normal behavior and what is not. This is a serious problem that parents face with America's teens. Several red flags that often exist in teens suffering clinical depression are:

- ☐ Personality changes, crying or sadness;

- ☐ Dropping grades;

- ☐ Difficulty in relationships;

- ☐ Running away from home;

- ☐ Changes in eating patterns;

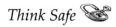

- ☐ Writing/talking about death;
- ☐ Talking about suicide;
- ☐ Low self-esteem;
- ☐ Other similar behaviors.

Again, these red flags are often overlooked because parents don't spend enough time with their teen to fully understand and/or recognize behavioral changes.

Suicide Intervention

When a teen's behavior is identified as a red flag, some form of intervention is necessary. The most important factor is open interaction between you and your teen — interaction in terms of talking *with* your teenager as opposed to talking *to* your teenager. The difference is that talking *to* the teenager is a one-way conversation. Talking *with* the teenager provides an opportunity for meaningful dialogue from which ideas and opinions are discussed. Additionally, it provides an opportunity to listen carefully, to assess, and reassure your love as the parent. Christine Taylor advises in her ***Ohio State Extension Fact Sheet*** that if a teen with depressive illness does not receive help, he or she may turn to suicide as an escape. Adding, four main danger signals of suicide are:

1) Threats or talk of killing oneself.

2) Preparing for death. Giving away prized possessions, making a will, farewell letters, or saying goodbye.

3) Talking like there is no hope for the future.

4) Acting or talking like not a single person cares. Completely giving up on self and others.

Teens exhibiting any suicide danger signals should be taken seriously and receive help from a qualified professional. Some resources are the **American Academy of Child & Adolescent Psychiatry** (www.aacap.org) and **Screening for Mental Health, Inc.** (www.mentalhealthscreening.org).

Chapter 4

BABYSITTERS

Guide for Parents

As a parent, the most important things in your life are your children. The act of entrusting their care, particularly infants and toddlers, to babysitters is a major event. Frequently, the babysitter cares for the child or children in your home. Thus a review of household conditions is important to ensure the babysitter is working in a safe environment. The following list contains items that should be in place at all times, but especially before asking someone to accept responsibility for your child's welfare in your home.

- ☐ House address numbers should be clearly visible from the street for emergency responders.

- ☐ Exterior lighting should be functional.

- ☐ Smoke alarms recently checked. Fire extinguishers recently charged.

- ☐ All firearms secured in a gun safe.

- ☐ Emergency phone list posted by each phone.

- ☐ All medicines should be secured.

- ☐ All doors and windows should have workable locks.

- ☐ Front door should have a viewer.

- ☐ In two-story homes, a fire escape ladder should be available on the second level.

- ☐ Electrical plugs, appliances, and cords should be secured.

- ☐ Household cleaners and solutions should be secured.

Additionally, you must leave clear, complete, and concise written instructions including the family name; children's names; house address with nearest cross street; where you will be and phone numbers; cell and pager numbers; the name and phone number of a trusted neighbor in case of an emergency; the name of the family doctor and directions to the nearest hospital emergency room; fire, police, and poison hot line; medications and how to administer them; and any special instructions.

Guide for Babysitters

If your teenager has recently taken a job as a babysitter, understand the enormous responsibility of this position. Your teen must care for and ensure the safety of a child or children. To prepare your teen for this responsibility, start by reiterating what is expected of them, and how they should carry out the expectations.

The first step is to take care of your teen's personal safety. Only allow them to take babysitting jobs from people you know or from those who are referred to your teen's service by a mutual acquaintance. Always get the name, address, and phone number of where your teen will be working, and also the time you can expect the job to end. When the job is complete, ask your teen to phone you for a ride or get an escort home from the employer. Never allow your teen to walk home alone in the dark without telling a trusted adult the route they plan to take, and the estimated arrival time. Make sure your teen knows the importance of always letting you know they are on the way home. And let your teen know that if the employer seems intoxicated, not to get in the car with them.

The next step is to ensure the safety of the children under your teen's care. Be sure he or she has an emergency contact information list, and if the employer does not have one prepared, then they should know to make one. This list should include the family name, children's names, house address and cross street, telephone number where the parents will be, a nearby neighbor's name and number, and the child's doctor's name and number. A signed medical release is also a good idea. To ensure your teen doesn't overlook any items, make a check-off list for them ahead of time. This way, if the parent calls on your teen's services again it will be easy to just update the list.

To make sure your teen is ready for babysitting responsibilities, review the following list of requirements with them, and make sure they know to do each of the items while on the job:

- ☐ Get written instructions on medications if they are required to give them to a child.

- ☐ Get a tour of the home. Determine off-limits areas for the children if there are any. Identify hazards like plastic bags, chemicals, and other dangers for a child.

- [ ] During the tour, check that all the windows and doors are locked. Ask the parent for a demonstration of how they work, and then try them.

- [ ] Tour outside to check water hazards such as pool or spa.

- [ ] Meet family pets.

- [ ] Find out the location of the smoke alarm.

- [ ] Visiting friends may distract your teen from their responsibility, so it is not a good idea to have visitors. If visitors are a must, clear them with the employer.

- [ ] If your teen answers the telephone, make sure they know not to tell the caller they are alone but take a message.

- [ ] If someone knocks, make sure your teen knows not to answer the front door. They should talk to the visitor through the door, but not tell them that they are alone.

- [ ] If they feel insecure at any point, tell them to call the police, and have their checklist handy so they can answer their questions.

- [ ] When the children go to bed, your teen should check on them every fifteen minutes or less.

- [ ] If children are up and about, let your teen know the importance of knowing where they are at all times, and to be particularly aware of silences.

- [ ] Make sure your teen monitors TV programs and movies, and only allow parentally approved viewing.

- [ ] Tell your teen never to leave the children alone. If they must leave the house, they should take the children.

- [ ] In the event of a fire, make sure your teen knows to get the children out and not to go back into the house. They should go to the predetermined nearby neighbors' house, and call 911 to report the fire.

Remember, a babysitter has an enormous responsibility, so always be sure your teen is prepared for the job.

Chapter 5 ON-LINE PARENTING

T he electronic age presents a particular need for involvement by parents with children and computers. Many web sites promote sexually explicit material, hate-oriented material, drug use, and bomb making. And the government has not been very effective, to date, at restricting access to these sites because courts have in the past, and will probably continue to be very sensitive to laws related to First Amendment concerns. What can you do as a parent to control the objectionable content viewed by your children on the Internet? Three things:

1) Supervise children while they're online.

2) Install filtering software to prevent objectionable material from getting through. If placed between the computer's web browser, such as Microsoft's Internet Explorer, or Netscape Navigator, or your ISP (Internet Service Provider, e.g. AOL, MSN, Prodigy, CompuServe, Earthlink), then objectionable words or images may be blocked. The drawback to filters is they often block harmless items due to software configurations and/or value judgments.

3) Install monitoring software, which reports on sites the user has visited.

The following ISP and/or software providers offer selections of filter products suitable for the entire family.

☐ America Online (AOL) is an ISP (Internet Service Provider). As a member of the service, AOL's Parental Controls allow you to designate different levels of access for each child:

- *Kids Only* (twelve and under): restricts children to certain areas on AOL and the Internet (when accessed through AOL).

- *Young Teen* (thirteen - fifteen): does not provide full access to content or interactive features.

- *Mature Teen* (sixteen - seventeen): Mature Teens can access all content on AOL and the Internet, except certain sites deemed for an adult (eighteen and over) audience.

☐ CyberPatrol, Version 6.2 can filter mail and block selected applications. An on-line list of objectionable websites is automatically updated. This software is available in Windows and Macintosh.

☐ Cybersitter 2000 (www.cybersitter.com) has an on-line list of objectionable web sites, which is automatically updated. It can filter mail, downloads, and custom word lists. It can also log activity.

☐ Cybersnoop (www.pearlsw.com) can filter objectionable web sites, e-mail, downloads, custom word lists, and also log activity.

☐ Net Nanny (www.netnanny.com) provides a list of objectionable web sites that is automatically updated. It filters custom word lists, sites labeled with some content ratings, and logs activity.

To choose the filter most suitable for your needs, examine the above web sites and compare the features. Many offer free trial offers, and P.C. Magazine (www.pcmag.com) periodically publishes reviews of filtering software and posts these reviews on-line.

Public libraries pose a significant concern in that they serve a diverse public, and therefore their rules of site access may be very liberal or unstructured. If your child's interest in visiting the library suddenly increases, take notice and question their increased interest.

Managing Internet Use[1]

For Parents

Talk with your children and reach agreement about the rules before you make the decision to go on-line in your home. Understand that by accessing the Internet, you enter a new world of responsibility as a parent. Control issues are very different and the skills required to protect children are new. Protecting children in the Internet environment is a combination of common sense, good parenting, teaching children the rules of computer safety, using the parental support tools available, and remembering that good parents are those who encourage and get involved with their children.

Strategies for Parents

- ☐ Set limits, or House Rules, for computer use.

- ☐ Parents and children should work together to set these House Rules.

- ☐ Place the computer in a family room with plenty of traffic, not behind closed doors.

- ☐ Express your interest in what the kids are doing and learning on the computer.

- ☐ Learn about the Internet with your children. If your children know more about the Internet than you do, let them be your guide.

- ☐ Manage their time on-line, and balance their lives between computer use and other activities.

- ☐ Use appropriate filters, and monitor on-line activity.

- ☐ Follow-up with children to determine whether they follow the House Rules.

Web Safety Tips for Children

Children must understand that the Internet allows people to communicate anonymously, and therefore, people can pretend to be whoever they want to be. People met on-line are strangers and not necessarily who they say they are. Additionally, the Internet contains information and views that may offend and upset them. To protect themselves, your children should:

- ☐ **ALWAYS** notify a parent if someone they have "met" on-line wants to meet in person.

- ☐ **ALWAYS** be themselves on-line, and never pretend to be anyone or anything they are not.

☐ **NEVER** give out personal information to others on the Internet, e.g. name, address, phone number, or a photograph.

☐ **ALWAYS** tell parents about anything they saw on the Internet that upsets or worries them.

☐ **NEVER** resond to an e-mail or instant message that makes you feel uncomfortable.

☐ **NEVER** give out passwords.

Warning Signals

Watch out for specific warning signs that may indicate your child has a problem with pornography on the Internet. Keep in mind that as a parent, you are looking for a trend; not jumping to conclusions at every little sign.

☐ Children hide computer CD's or disks.

☐ Children quickly change the computer screen when you enter the room.

☐ Children spend a lot of time on the Internet, or are on-line late into the night.

☐ Changes in behavior, for example, secretiveness, inappropriate sexual knowledge, mention of adults you don't know, or new sleeping problems.

☐ Your credit card statement lists phone charges that identify themselves as "websites." Pornographers avoid providing their names.

The Internet offers children many opportunities for learning, constructive entertainment, and personal growth. At the same time, you must be concerned about the risks your children face on-line. Your challenge as a parent is to educate yourself and your children about how to use the Internet safely.

1 *Surf Control White Paper* http//:www.surfcontrol.com

Chapter 6

COLLEGE CONSIDERATIONS

Choosing the right institution for higher learning is often based on several factors, including cost, location, academics, and competition. Although safety is usually not a primary factor in choosing a college, it should be taken into account. As many students have never been away from home, evaluation of safety and security is very important in the college selection process. And many campuses emphasize safety in their recruitment materials. When your student starts thinking about a particular school, plan a visit to the law enforcement group.

A college campus is generally policed by a formal group, such as campus security or law enforcement, and is required to maintain campus crime statistics. During this college visit, inquire about the school's recent crime reports, their crime investigation process, and the common outcomes of their inquiries. Request crime prevention information, and also material related to self-protection and theft prevention programs. At minimum, the institution should offer brochures that address these issues. Your on-campus college student must focus on protecting themselves in their new environment with consideration for things like locks, key control, personal property, and personal risk.

Sending children to college, for many families, means they are leaving home for the first time. They will be alone, making their own decisions, and parents can often do little more than hope for the best. But parents who take an active approach to teaching safety help their children to be better prepared for making the right decisions when they are on their own. Additional personal safety precautions, such as personal defense weapons and apartment security, are covered in later chapters.

Section Two – Safety Precautions for Women

- CHAPTER 7 - COLLEGE CONSIDERATIONS
- CHAPTER 8 - RAPE DEFENSE
- CHAPTER 9 - DOMESTIC VIOLENCE

Introduction

Most women know that, as a gender, they must be more concerned with their personal safety than men, although the number of victimizations of women is nearly even with the number of men. In 2002, the US Bureau of Justice Statistics recorded almost 5.5 million personal victimizations. These were victims of crimes of violence such as rape/sexual assault, robbery, and other minor assaults. Slightly over 2.5 million, or half of these cases were females, according to the Personal Crimes 2002 report from the US Department of Justice Statistics. For detailed information regarding the victimization rates please refer to the Table 1 - Victimization by Age, Gender and Type of Crime.

But women must be more concerned because they can be viewed as an easier target then men, perhaps because they are smaller in stature, lighter in weight, and stereotypical less violent in nature. If a predator has the option of attacking and robbing a man or a woman, chances are he will choose the woman every time. And the nature of crimes committed against women is often more severe and more emotionally damaging, such as rape and sexual assault.

This entire section has been devoted to the extra precautions women need to take in college, when dating, and even when their mate or intimate partner becomes abusive. These precautions will help ease anxiety, especially for women who live alone or travel alone. And for those women who are in abusive relationships, this section contains information they can use to get out of the situation. When women use these safety precautions, they empower themselves with independence, security, and awareness.

Victimization by Age, Gender and Type of Crime

Number of victimizations and victimization rates for persons age 12 and over, by type of crime and gender of victims

Rate per 1,000 persons age 12 and over

Type of crime	Both genders		Male		Female	
	Number	Rate	Number	Rate	Number	Rate
All personal crimes	**5,496,810**	**23.7**	**2,927,520**	**26.1**	**2,569,300**	**21.5**
Crimes of violence	5,341,410	23.1	2,857,930	25.5	2,483,480	20.8
Completed violence	1,753,090	7.6	816,240	7.3	936,850	7.8
Attempted/threatened violence	3,588,320	15.5	2,041,690	18.2	1,546,630	13.0
Rape/Sexual assault	247,730	1.1	31,640	0.3	216,090	1.8
Rape/Attempted rape	167,860	0.7	22,610	0.2 *	145,240	1.2
Rape	90,390	0.4	4,100	0.0 *	86,290	0.7
Attempted rape/a	77,470	0.3	18,520	0.2 *	58,950	0.5
Sexual assault/b	79,870	0.3	9,030	0.1 *	70,840	0.6
Robbery	512,490	2.2	323,530	2.9	188,960	1.6
Completed/property taken	385,880	1.7	237,350	2.1	148,530	1.2
With injury	169,980	0.7	102,860	0.9	67,130	0.6
Without injury	215,890	0.9	134,490	1.2	81,400	0.7
Attempted to take property	126,610	0.5	86,180	0.8	40,430	0.3
With injury	42,600	0.2	31,470	0.3	11,130	0.1 *
Without injury	84,020	0.4	54,710	0.5	29,300	0.2 *
Assault	4,581,190	19.8	2,502,760	22.3	2,078,440	17.4
Aggravated	990,110	4.3	588,430	5.2	401,670	3.4
With injury	316,260	1.4	166,930	1.5	149,330	1.3
Threatened with weapon	673,850	2.9	421,510	3.8	252,350	2.1
Simple	3,591,090	15.5	1,914,320	17.1	1,676,760	14.0
With minor injury	906,580	3.9	405,670	3.6	500,910	4.2
Without injury	2,684,510	11.6	1,508,650	13.4	1,175,860	9.9
Purse snatching/Pocket picking	155,400	0.7	69,590	0.6	85,810	0.7
Population age 12 and over	231,589,260	...	112,241,930	...	119,347,330	...

Note: Detail may not add to total shown because of rounding.
*Estimate is based on about 10 or fewer sample cases.
...Not applicable.
a/Includes verbal threats of rape.
b/Includes threats.

Chapter 7

COLLEGE CONSIDERATIONS

Especially for Women

During college years, women may experience a wide range of unwanted sexual experiences. And it is generally accepted that these unwanted experiences become criminal at the point a victim says "no" and the "no" is ignored. These experiences may occur with a stranger, a friend, a boyfriend, a fellow student, a professor, or someone met in a social setting. And the experience may occur on or off campus, in the residence hall, at a place of employment, or even while jogging among other people. These experiences can happen while awake, asleep, unconscious, or drunk. Therefore, as a woman, you need to keep your personal safety in mind at all times.

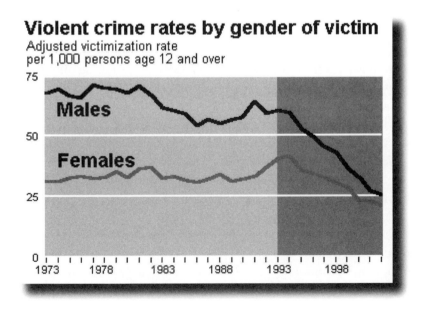

Violent crime rates by gender of victim
Adjusted victimization rate
per 1,000 persons age 12 and over

Date Rape

September 2002

The U.S. Attorney General announced the arrest of 115 individuals in eighty-four cities for selling date rape drugs over the Internet.

Sexual predators use a variety of different drugs, such as GHB, GBL, and 1,4 Butanediol (1,4BD and also known as "G" and "Liquid X"). These drugs are commonly referred to as "date rape drugs" because they act on the central nervous system as depressants. Virtually undetectable, these drugs are odorless and colorless, but extremely potent. Their side effects include drowsiness, dizziness, loss of consciousness, loss of inhibition, and memory impairment. Higher doses of these drugs may cause seizures, severe respiratory depression, coma, and death.

Predators administer these illicit drugs by putting them in the beverages of unsuspecting victims at parties, bars, nightclubs, or other social settings. Because these drugs are colorless, tasteless, and odorless, the victim has no way of knowing if their drink will cause severe impairment and defenselessness. After the drugs are ingested, the victim is at the mercy of the predator(s). Significant amnesia may result, causing the victim to be unclear on what, if any, crime was committed. Additionally, victims of drug-facilitated sexual assault cannot protect themselves from HIV, other sexually transmitted diseases, or pregnancy.

Defenses

Drink responsibly. Know your tolerance for alcohol and avoid intoxication. Intoxication lowers inhibitions that may increase risk taking and bad decisions, among others. If excessive alcohol consumption is likely, take a non-drinker along to see that you return home safely.

Besides making you more vulnerable for sexual predators, drinking can be dangerous in other ways. Each year over a thousand students die from alcohol-related accidents. Half a million students are injured in a year from alcohol-related situations, and nearly a hundred thousand women are victims of alcohol-related rapes or sexual assaults.

Be cautious of strangers buying your drinks. Accepting drinks from strangers creates a significant weakness in personal safety, and sets up an opportunity for a predator to poison you.

Drink Safe Technology 2002 has developed two methods for detecting drugs in drinks. The first method is a drink safe kit, which contain strips that change colors when introduced to a spiked drink. These strips are easy to use and the test takes only seconds to perform. Detection strips indicate the introduction of a foreign substance into the drink, but they are not infallible. They should be considered only one component of an overall prevention plan. Other components include keeping your drink with you at all times, if possible, and agreeing with your friends to watch one another's drink. If you're seated at a table, try to keep one person at the table at all times to prevent drink doctoring while you're gone.

Drink test coasters are the second recent development in drink testing. Like the strips, these coasters can identify if a drink has been spiked. They have two active test areas on the bottom corners of the 4 x 4 coaster, and complete instructions for use are printed on the back.

Drink safe tests are new to the marketplace and thus have no measurable reliability factor, so until further data is available don't rely on theses devices completely. At this point, they should be considered for their potential deterrent value.

Rape of College Women

A joint research report by the United States Department of Justice, the National Institute of Justice, and the Bureau of Justice Statistics (BJS) on "The Sexual Victimization of College Women" (12-2000), contributes significant information about the occurrence of on-campus sex crimes. This report concluded that three percent of female college students will be raped or will suffer an attempted rape every six months. Extrapolating that number over the entire college career equals a staggering 350 incidents of rape per academic year on a campus of 10,000 women.

Prevention Strategies

☐ Awareness. Always be aware of where you are and what's going on around you.

☐ Body Language. Walk with a determined step, stand straight up, and swing your arms.

☐ Walk with a friend, if possible.

☐ Have your car keys in your hand well before you get to the vehicle.

☐ Park your car with darkness in mind if it is late in the day. Park under light poles near your exit.

☐ When jogging, go with a friend whenever possible, and plan your route. If you're alone, tell someone your route and expected return time.

☐ Always carry a whistle. Keep it handy.

☐ Consider self-defense training classes, but keep in mind this requires a long-term commitment with regular practice.

Stalkers

Stalking is also addressed in the aforementioned BJS Research Report. Thirteen percent of sampled college women were victimized by stalkers as defined by, "experiencing repeated, obsessive, and frightening behavior that made the victim afraid or concerned for her safety." The most common form of stalking was by telephone, and the second most common was by following or waiting around for the victim. In over fifteen percent of occurrences the stalker threatened or attempted to harm the victim, and in over ten percent of occurrences, the stalker forced or attempted sexual contact. Typically, stalking behavior lasted sixty days per incident.

Nothing feels more disturbing than being stalked. Your personal life is invaded by an undesired person who imposes emotional and psychological trauma. Besides invading your privacy, stalkers take away your freedom, disrupt your telephone activity, and may force you into a job change, dropping classes, changing majors, and changing your personal habits because of their presence in your life. Victims worry about both real and imaginary dangers, and they agonize over how to stop their aggressor.

Prevention Strategies

☐ Upon recognition of unwanted contact, communicate your lack of interest with firm, short, and to-the-point responses.

☐ Your first response should be the only response you give the stalker. Engaging them in conversation translates to encouragement in their minds, and will ultimately prolong their persistence.

☐ Do not acknowledge electronic mail from the stalker. Do not open it; just delete it.

☐ Get an answering machine for your telephone and monitor your calls before picking up. Do not accept or answer the stalker's calls.

☐ Avoid the stalker. This may mean personal sacrifices in your activities.

☐ Involve law enforcement by reporting the incidents.

Chapter 8 R APE D EFENSE

Rape is an act of violent hostility to achieve power. Rape and having sex are not the same. Rape is a frightening experience with life-long traumatic ramifications. Rape affects everyone regardless of age, sex or ethnicity. All women are potential victims of a sexual assault. Recognizing this and becoming psychologically sensitive to the issue may reduce the likelihood of becoming a victim. Psychologically sensitive means to accept the fact that you are a potential victim, to prepare for an attack through rape prevention education, and to develop an awareness of locations and situations where rape is likely to occur and to avoid them.

When thinking about rape defense, your first thoughts may lead to chemical mace, pepper spray, stun guns, handguns, or martial arts. Each of these defense mechanisms will be discussed later, but rape defense actually begins long before any of these tools becomes necessary.

Many Victims Know Their Rapist

A high percentage of rapes occur in dating situations, meaning that the victim knows her attacker before the actual attack occurs. Maybe the attacker is an acquaintance, a friend, a classmate, or even a date. But regardless of whether a victim knows the attacker, or if the victim has agreed to spend time with her attacker, the fact remains that everyone has a right to refuse unwanted sexual contact. No one has the right to force sexual contact on another person, even someone they've had sex with before. Sex is not something that is owned, or something required as payback for a good time. A person who insists on sex in these circumstances is looking for power and control. Beware of these kinds of relationships.

You can prevent date rape situations by setting prerequisites for a first date, such as having a say in where you are going and whom you will be with. Avoid private settings until you know the person better. Prearrange alternate transportation should you need to leave the date. Carry emergency funds just in case. Always let others know whom you are with, where you are going, and what you will be doing. Above all, trust your intuition. If a situation doesn't feel right, do something about it. Take charge, be aggressive, and get out of the situation. When denying sex in dating situations, communication must be clear and assertive. Don't expect your date to guess what you mean. Mean what you say and say what you mean, firmly. No means no. Do not send mixed signals.

Remember, alcohol and/or drugs impair the ability to think and act. This impairment makes the rapist's actions easier to carry out. Always exercise prudence with intoxicating drugs, and never invite a person who you met in a bar to be alone with you in your home.

Be alert to unexpected conversation about sex or dirty jokes. If you feel uncomfortable, let the date know right away it's gone too far. Recognize this as an opportunity to be assertive and get out of the situation before it gets worse. If the date's sexual advances continue, delay by saying something like you need another hour or two to get to know each other or assure that on the next date you will do everything he/she wants. Seek to escape, attract assistance, or talk your way out.

Attacks in the Home

Protection from sexual assault requires constant awareness of yourself, your surroundings, and an attacker's likely strategies. Awareness is a learned skill, thus it takes practice and a little time but it can be a lifesaver. Over time, with practice, awareness can become a habit. Predators survive on surprise of the unaware, but by being aware and projecting an "in control" presence, attacks may be averted. So develop a habit of paying attention at all times to whatever is going on around you.

The following is excerpted from the *San Jose Mercury News*:

The story lead, "Rape Linked to Sex Predator," follows with: A sexual predator who often poses as a plumber has assaulted at least 30 Bay Area women since April 2000 with the most recent attack when he raped a woman in her home after subduing her with a stun gun. The victims range in age from 17-65. For months, the man exposed himself or groped women in apartment complexes or carports. The assailant recently posed as a plumber to check the water pipes. Upon return, he gained entrance, shocked the woman repeatedly with a stun gun then raped her.

The attacker most commonly posed as a plumber, handyman, or construction worker and tried to talk his way into women's apartments or condos. He approached some women in apartment complex parking lots, many of which were upscale or gated complexes. He made contact at the door, said he is a plumber and the maintenance man sent him to check on things and women let him in.

As illustrated in the aforementioned newspaper account, many rapes occur in the home. Whether you own or rent your residence does not affect elements of crime prevention, besides the fact that renters almost always need permission to alter the premises with supplemental locks or hardware.

Safety at Home

A number of factors, physical and environmental, significantly affect security of the residence. If affordable, a security consultant should conduct a home security survey. This survey will identify strengths and weaknesses, while taking into account environmental and physical influences (see Chapter 19 page 147 on Home Security for a complete Home Security Checklist). Some physical and environmental issues may be easier for the homeowner than renters to achieve. However, you should not hesitate to notify a property owner of a safety-security issue to make them aware of the situation.

Following are precautions and security measures for the home:

- ☐ Prior to moving into a previously occupied dwelling, change the locks.

- ☐ Upgrade or add a dead bolt lock to exterior doors.

- ☐ Add a peephole if none exists.

- ☐ Ensure all entrances are well-lit at night.

- ☐ Keep the garage door down and locked at all times.

- ☐ Consider using multiple timers for lights, radio, etc.

- ☐ If you arrive home and find suspicious circumstances, do not enter. Go to a neighbor's house and call police.

☐ Keep drapes and shades closed at night.

☐ If you hear a prowler, turn on all lights and call the police.

☐ Do not hide extra house keys. Instead, leave a key with a trusted neighbor for emergencies.

☐ When on vacation, cancel newspapers and have the post office hold the mail.

☐ Door chains are ineffective. Utilize the peephole to identify callers.

☐ Do not allow children to open the door.

☐ Ask for identification of all service personnel before opening the door. If in an apartment, call the office and verify the person.

☐ Never allow a stranger into your home.

☐ Keep all doors and windows closed and locked when you're away. This includes short trips to the store, etc.

☐ Keep shrubs and bushes neatly trimmed to avert concealment.

☐ Get in and out of common apartment laundry rooms as quickly as possible.

☐ Exercising in apartment facilities should be in the company of another, if possible.

☐ Install an alarm system with a panic feature. The panic feature is an excellent tool for coming and going to carports, parking, etc. Vehicle alarms have a similar feature; however, most people are desensitized to car alarms.

Other precautions:

☐ Always walk or jog with a friend and stay in well-lit areas.

☐ Avoid shortcuts that take you away from a well-traveled path.

☐ When street walking, avoid walking close to doorways, shrubs, and places that offer concealment.

☐ Walk against the traffic unless it is threatening.

☐ If a car stops and asks a question, stay away from the car.

☐ Keep keys in your hand with the longest key held tightly and extending outward for use as a defensive weapon. Additionally, it eliminates fumbling for keys to enter the residence.

☐ If you suspect you're being followed, go to an open business or a fire or police department for safety.

☐ Avoid hitchhiking.

Precautions in and around a vehicle:

☐ Service your vehicles regularly to prevent unexpected break-downs. Have fluids, tires, and belts checked. Always keep gas level above a ¼ tank.

☐ Plan ahead. Have your keys out and ready as you approach your parked vehicle. Look at and around the vehicle, and quickly glance into the back seat before entering.

☐ Keep car doors locked at all times.

☐ If your car is being serviced, leave only the car key. NEVER leave home keys.

☐ Anticipate darkness when parking. Select a parking spot that will be well-lit upon return.

☐ Be alert to vehicles parked in your vicinity, particularly vans because they are frequently involved in abductions.

☐ In stop-and-go traffic, leave enough room between you and the car ahead so you can get out of the lane quickly, if necessary.

☐ Do not lower your car windows enough for someone to reach in.

☐ If someone signals that something is wrong with your vehicle, do not stop until they are out of the area. Their signal may be a ruse to get you to stop.

Sexual Assaults

An intended rape victim has three options: appealing to the attacker, resisting the attacker, or submitting to the attacker.

Appealing to the attacker: The objective of appealing to the attacker is to think and talk your way out of the situation. Strategies that you might employ are:

☐ Try to calm the attacker and persuade him not to continue.

☐ Claim to be sick, pregnant, or carrying a disease.

☐ Try to divert him. Pretend to faint. Act insane.

☐ Lie to him. Tell him you expect someone to return soon.

Resisting the attacker: Resisting is intended to injure the attacker at least long enough to escape. Resistance is a personal decision, and you must weigh the probability of success, opportunity for success, and mental attitude for success, because once your resistance begins the attacker is likely to retaliate with force. Common ways to resist include:

☐ Make a ruckus, yell, or scream in an attempt to distract the attacker and escape. Words like, "fire," and, "police," might draw attention. But the effectiveness of yelling depends on someone hearing you.

☐ Fight back (mental attitude). You must not be afraid to hurt an attacker. Kicks, blows, and actions must apply physical pain and buy enough time for your escape.

☐ Martial arts. Self-defense skills require a significant amount of dedication to acquire and to maintain proficiency.

☐ Weapons. Carrying weapons such as guns, knives, mace, or pepper spray can be dangerous if proficiency is not maintained. Additionally, the attacker may turn a weapon against you. Most, if not all, of these weapons are regulated and require license to carry.

Submission: Always remember your primary concern should be your safety, and at times you won't have the opportunity to resist. If you feel you have a low probability for successful resistance or violence toward an aggressor, then no one can tell you whether you should submit or fight back. Each situation is unique and depends on several variables. Your best defenses are to be aware, to know your options, and to be prepared to execute your choice of options very quickly.

Rape Trauma

Rape victims often exhibit significant emotional responses such as irritability, crying, inability to sleep, denial, anger, grief, and depression. Professional counseling should be arranged to deal with these issues. Rape Crisis Centers are in most cities and provide expert assistance.

The support of family and friends is also very important for someone who has been sexually assaulted. Family and friends must realize that they are also likely to experience significant emotional reactions because supporting someone who has been sexually assaulted can be very difficult. Professional guidance for those providing support is also very important.

Police and Prosecution

Unfortunately, rape is among the leaders of unreported crimes. Some estimate that over half of rapes go unreported to police. Clearly fear, humiliation, and embarrassment may be possible reasons for keeping an incident secret, but rape victims must realize that many rapists are repeat offenders, and reporting rape will help prevent future rapes. By working with the information from reported rapes and their surrounding circumstances, personal safety awareness can improve. If you have been raped you must report the incident as soon as possible, and if someone you know has been raped, you must encourage and support her to do the same.

A successful prosecution of the offender depends in large part on the victim's ability to put the rapist at the scene of the crime. This is accomplished through details from the victim and clinical evidence taken by medical personnel. Therefore, the victim must inform police of all details of the attack, and of anything unusual about the attacker. This includes what the attacker said and how it was said, and showing the police all bruises or injuries from the attack, no matter how small. Remember that some bruises may appear in the following day or days.

In regard to physical evidence, after the rape has occurred the victim must not shower, douche, change clothing, or disturb the assault scene. Medical personnel will take semen smears and document observations for trial purposes. The victim's clothing will also be taken for evidence to associate the attacker to the crime. Information the police will need to capture the rapist will include:

- ☐ Type of vehicle, license, make, model, color; may be a bicycle or other type of transportation;

- ☐ Race;

☐ Age, weight, height;

☐ Hair color and characteristics;

☐ Eye color;

☐ Marks, scars, tattoos;

☐ Facial hair;

☐ Other distinctions – rings, necklaces, piercings.

Chapter 9

DOMESTIC VIOLENCE

Reports show that one in three women in the United States is abused. And if these reports are even nearly accurate, they are staggering. But perhaps even more staggering is the fact that the woman is likely to return to an abusive environment an average of seven times.

In an abusive relationship, the abuser may employ physical violence, emotional and verbal abuse, threats, or intimidation and isolation to keep power and control over his or her partner. The following points describe these behaviors in more detail:

- ☐ **Physical Violence.** The abuser, most often a male, beats the female. Many times a drunken argument precedes the beating, and injuries include bruises, cuts, black eye/s, broken bones, and worse.

- ☐ **Emotional and Verbal Abuse.** The abuser degrades his partner with put downs, public humiliation, and name-calling.

- ☐ **Isolation**. Abusers are generally extremely jealous. And their jealousy is demonstrated by insisting the partner disassociate with family and friends.

- ☐ **Threats and Intimidation.** Threats of violence, of suicide, or of taking the children away are common tactics used by domestic abusers.

According to the government publication, ***Domestic Violence Awareness Handbook,*** the existence of emotional and verbal abuse, attempts to isolate, and threats and intimidation within a relationship may indicate that physical abuse is to follow.

The Cycle of Violence

Experts say the cycle of violence, generally present in a violent relationship, consists of a tension building stage, a violent episode stage, and a honeymoon or reconciliation stage.

Nancy Wilson, a Domestic Violence Educator, interviewed August 26, 2002 in ***The Mountain Democrate Newspaper***, describes the tension building stage as the time when the woman is walking on eggshells, trying not to upset the balance of civility in the house. She will make sure the laundry is folded just right, the kids are quiet, and the house is clean.

But none of these activities will make a difference, according to Ken Stefan, the executive director of the El Dorado County Women's Center. He asserts that when the situation is going to erupt, it will, regardless of how perfect the victim has tried to be. Any small or insignificant event can set off a domestic abuser. When a meal is a little burnt or a long line at the grocery store delays dinner, it can start the second stage, which is violence.

In many cases, the victims report a perfect life…except for the beatings. Besides her broken ribs, fractures, cuts, bruises, and black eyes, she believes her marriage is perfect. Sometimes, women in abusive relationships go so far as to plan the violence, according to Wilson. For example, they set it off by doing something to aggravate their partner on a Friday night in hopes that the bruises will be gone by Monday morning.

The honeymoon or reconciliation stage is the point the batterer feels sorry and remorseful. This stage is marked with flowers, sweet words, and promises not to repeat the violence—perhaps even a promise to go to counseling. These promises give the victim hope, but rarely mean anything to the abuser. And so, the cycle continues with the batterer in total control over the victim with little, if any change.

Incidents of domestic violence involve family secrets. The victim usually begins to believe the demeaning things the batterer says about them are true. Or the victim is fearful that the beating she will get as punishment for reporting the incident will be worse than what she has already experienced.

An example of these factors in action is clearly demonstrated in a local police blotter entry that read, "Domestic violence/assault with a deadly weapon. A twenty-three-year-old male stabbed his girlfriend three times in the arm and punched her in the face while they were driving local streets. The woman told her family about the incident, but did not report it to the police. A family member reported the incident to police on her behalf whereupon a countywide search for her boyfriend was initiated."

The Batterer

Until the batterer comes to grips with the idea that he does not have the right to control another person and learns how to control his anger appropriately, the cycle of violence will continue. Domestic abusers need help to recognize that their behavior must change. Intervention often comes from the justice system through court referrals to treatment programs. Without intervention, the abusive relationship could end in tragedy.

Court Process and Legal Terms

A domestic violence case often begins with law enforcement intervention. Some terms and process explanation may be helpful to understand how a case moves through the legal system. Not all states have an identical process, but they should share similarities.

☐ **Defendant:** A person charged with a crime.

☐ **Arraignment:** The first time a defendant appears in court.

- ✦ Charges are read.

- ✦ Judge asks the defendant if they can afford an attorney.

- ✦ If the defendant cannot afford one, an attorney is appointed.

- ✦ The next court date is set.

☐ **Court Review:** The judge, district attorney, and defense attorney try to reach an agreement regarding the case.

- ✦ May take more than one court hearing.

- ✦ Victim does not have to attend.

- ✦ If the case does not settle, it goes forward. In major crimes, a preliminary hearing may follow.

☐ **Preliminary Hearing:** A court hearing where evidence regarding the case is presented.

✦ Subpoenas (written orders to appear in court) are issued to witnesses and the victim.

✦ Victim may testify.

✦ Police officers who took a report or witnessed the incident testify.

✦ If a subpoenaed person does not come to court a warrant may be issued for their arrest.

✦ The judge will hear the evidence and decide if there is enough for a trial.

✦ If sufficient evidence, a trial date is set.

☐ **Jury Trial:** The case is presented to a jury.

✦ Generally, a group of twelve, but may be fewer people.

✦ Victim testifies.

✦ Officers who filed the report testify.

✦ Other witnesses including family or neighbors may testify.

✦ Jury decides if the defendant is guilty or not.

✦ If the jury finds the defendant guilty, the case may go to a probation department for a sentencing report.

☐ **Probation Report:** A report written by a probation officer regarding the defendant's case. A sentencing recommendation to the judge is included.

✦ The report may include a victim's statement.

☐ **Restitution:** Money the defendant may be ordered to pay the victim for losses related to the crime.

☐ **Judgment and Sentence:** The judge sentences the defendant.

- ✦ May involve jail time.

- ✦ May include mandatory attendance in programs such as men's alternative to abusive patterns or anger management programs.

Recognizing Signs/ Symptoms of Domestic Violence

Violence is a learned behavior. Often signs can be detected in the young by their behavior toward other children, which may appear as bullying or acting out violent interactions of adults in his/her home environment. Other signs or symptoms of violence may include:

- ☐ Someone who is afraid of his/her partner. This could result from physical, emotional, and verbal abuse, or threats and intimidation in the relationship.

- ☐ Constantly apologizing for his/her partner's behavior. This could result from low self-esteem due to emotional and verbal abuse in the relationship.

- ☐ Bruises indicating physical abuse.

- ☐ The person works, but has no spending money for beverages, lunch, etc. This could indicate isolation abuse.

- ☐ Lack of freedom to do things outside the home. This behavior could result from isolation abuse.

Breaking the Cycle of Violence

The domestic violence cycle is unlikely to change absent intervention. Perhaps the short-term answer for intervention is an effective law enforcement action, e.g., arrest of abusers when a law has been broken. Jailing the offender at least creates an opportunity to get the offender:

- ☐ Punished;

- ☐ On probation with court supervision including in-home inspections and follow-up;

- ☐ Or referred for professional help.

Long-term answers to domestic abuse include education of the problem, development of prevention programs, and other social assistance facilities, such as shelters for families in distress. Most, if not all, states have a domestic violence prevention coalition, association, or agency for assistance.

The National Domestic Violence Hotline is a federal organization that can be reached at **1.800.799.SAFE.** Other resources may be found on the web by searching, *"preventing domestic violence."*

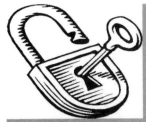

Section Three – Safety Precautions for the Elderly

- CHAPTER 10 - CRIMES AGAINST THE ELDERLY
- CHAPTER 11 - FINANCIAL (FIDUCIARY) ABUSE

Introduction

As people age, their vulnerability naturally increases. They become physically weak, forgetful, confused, and unaware of their surroundings. They may also become physically ill, or unable to take care of themselves. In some cases, especially after the death of a spouse, an elderly person may become lonely, depressed, or dependent on an unrelated third party for care. All these factors make elderly people easy prey.

Retirees may also start to worry about their finances and their long-term care. These concerns may influence them into poor decisions, or even to act out of desperation. And opportunistic criminals prey on these vulnerabilities. So when the elderly people you love start to show signs of increased vulnerability, you must take extra precautions to ensure their safety.

Chapter 10

CRIMES AGAINST THE ELDERLY

By the year 2030, an estimated sixty-six million people, or twenty-two percent of the population, will be in the age group of sixty-five and over, and those eighty-five years or older are the fastest growing group. As people age, they inevitably become more vulnerable to unscrupulous people. Already, recognition of elder abuse, neglect, and exploitation of the elderly in America represents an alarming trend. Seniors are victimized by their relatives, caregivers, con artists, telemarketers, investment groups, and predatory lenders, among others.

Elder Abuse

An accurate rate of incidence of elder abuse is difficult to determine; however, studies suggest occurrences are widespread. In part, the occurrence of elder abuse is hard to measure because it is largely hidden in domestic settings. Additionally, elderly people are in many cases entirely dependent on the abuser, and therefore reluctant to discuss the issue. One thing is certain, domestic elder abuse reports have increased steadily in the past several years. If the current rates of increase in the number of reports continue, the number of domestic elder abuse reports nationwide could be astounding.

From the national perspective, Louisiana Senator Breaux reported in his Elder Justice Proposal of 2002 Executive Summary, "There are between 500,000 and five million seniors who are abused in this country every year. Despite the dearth of data, experts agree that we have only seen the tip of the iceberg. Eighty-four percent of all cases are never even reported." Senator Breaux's report also states, "Congressional action remains elusive and not one single federal employee works full-time on elder abuse, neglect and exploitation issues."

Currently, state definitions of elder abuse vary considerably from one jurisdiction to another, in terms of what abuse, neglect, or exploitation is. Generally, three basic categories of elder abuse exist: domestic elder abuse, institutional elder abuse, and self-abuse.

Domestic elder abuse refers to any of several forms of cruelty or rough treatment of an older person by someone who has a relationship with the elderly person in the victim's own home or in the home of a caregiver. While the definitions differ, most jurisdictions collect statistical data on five types of domestic elder abuse. These five types are:

Physical Abuse, including but not limited to:

☐ Beatings;

☐ Unreasonable physical constraint;

☐ Prolonged deprivation of food or water

Sexual Abuse:

☐ Any absence of consent regarding sexual contact.

Psychological Abuse:

☐ Verbal assaults, threats, or harassment;

☐ Subjecting a person to fear, isolation, or serious emotional distress;

☐ Withholding emotional support;

☐ Confinement.

Financial (Fiduciary) Abuse:

☐ Theft;

☐ Embezzlement;

☐ Misuse of funds or property;

☐ Extortion;

☐ Fraud.

Neglect:

- ☐ Failure to assist in personal hygiene;

- ☐ Failure to provide clothing/shelter;

- ☐ Failure to provide medical care;

- ☐ Abandonment.

Institutional abuse refers to any of the above forms of abuse that occur in residential facilities. These facilities include nursing homes, group homes, or board and care facilities. Institutional abuse is committed by persons who have a legal or contractual obligation to provide elderly victims with care protection.

Elder self-abuse relates to harm or neglect, directed toward oneself. Harm or neglect may be recognized by physical indicators such as:

- ☐ Unkempt or dirty hair;

- ☐ Malnourished or dehydrated;

- ☐ Patches of hair missing;

- ☐ Soiled clothing or bed;

- ☐ Foul odor;

- ☐ Cuts, pinch marks, lacerations, or punctures;

- ☐ Unexplained bruises or welts;

- ☐ Burns;

- ☐ Injuries inconsistent with their explanation.

Self-neglect or self-abuse usually occurs as a result of physical or mental impairment. Also, social isolation may contribute to either neglect or abuse.

Elder abuse is not always a crime. Disrespect or rudeness may be distasteful but may not meet the requirements of a crime. Certainly, most physical, sexual, financial, or material abuses are considered criminal. In some circumstances, emotional abuse and neglect cases are subject to criminal prosecution, although they are often more difficult to prosecute.

Abusers of the Elderly

As Senator Breaux pointed out in his Elder Justice Proposal of 2002 Executive Summary, other family violence issues, such as domestic violence and child abuse, show that abuse, neglect, and exploitation require a multi-faceted solution. But while these other types of abuse have been recognized and receive sizable federal funding, elder abuse remains under-researched, under-reported, and under-funded.

Because these crimes are under-researched and under-reported, only a partial snapshot exists of who the elder abusers are. Utilizing data from 1994, the emerging picture in domestic settings indicate perpetrators of elder abuse as follows:

Adult Children	35.0%
Grandchildren	5.9%
Spouse	13.4%
Sibling	2.9%
Other Relatives	13.6%
Service Provider	6.2%
Friend/Neighbor	5.2%
All Others	10.3%
Unknown	7.4%

This, and associated research, also indicate that abusers:

☐ Are often related to the victim, and are usually adult children or spouses.

☐ May have problems such as drug and/or alcohol abuse.

The Victims

☐ Almost two-thirds are women;

☐ Are about 80 years of age;

☐ Usually live with the abuser.

Causes of Domestic Elder Abuse

Although the existing amount of knowledge on the subject is limited, a combination of psychological, social, and economic factors of both the victim and perpetrators are likely responsible. These factors include:

Stress of the caregiver:

☐ Shortage of money – either caregiver or elderly person;

☐ Unemployment;

☐ Inadequate coping skills, e.g. unable to deal with elderly person's memory loss and/or capacity to think or react.

Impairment of dependent elderly people:

☐ Severely disabled;

☐ Increased dependency on provider.

Cycle of Violence:

☐ Violence is seen as an acceptable way to solve problems.

☐ Many perpetrators repeat abusive behavior.

Personal problems of abusers:

☐ Adult children who abuse elderly people frequently have problems with mental and emotional disorders, alcoholism, and drug addictions.

☐ Dependence on the elderly person that results in abuse for money, among other reasons.

Preventing Elder Abuse

Domestic

Elder abuse is extremely complex and many factors contribute to its occurrence. But significant research efforts have been virtually absent from the agenda in this country. To develop better means for prevention and protection, research priorities must include national incidence and prevalence studies.

Until such studies provide another approach, the best way to make sure an elderly person is provided for is to plan ahead. By understanding the aging process, seniors, their family members, and friends can prepare for the physical and emotional changes, and make plans accordingly.

Long-Term Care

If or when long-term care is required, use the following criteria to assess the quality of care the person receives:

☐ Check on your aging friend or relative often.

☐ Are they getting quality care?

☐ Are they satisfied with the care?

☐ Listen to complaints carefully.

☐ Assist with resolving complaints.

☐ If unable to resolve a complaint, contact the long-term care ombudsman.

☐ If abuse is suspected, contact the local long-term care ombudsman or law enforcement immediately.

☐ Pay particular attention to the possibility of over-medicating. Some indicators include unsteadiness or frequent falls. Over-mediation may be used to control the elderly person by keeping them inactive.

Chapter 11 FINANCIAL / FIDUCIARY ABUSE

Financial abuse of elderly and dependent adults includes theft, embezzlement, misuse of funds or property, extortion, and fraud. The victims of this type of abuse are predominately females age seventy-five and older, and they are often reluctant to tell anyone because of embarrassment or dependency on the predator.

In this context, financial abuse is using an elderly person's money or assets contrary to their wishes, needs, best interests, or for the personal gain of the abuser. Some examples of financial abuse include, taking money or items from the elderly person's home or bank accounts; selling or transferring the elderly person's property against his/her wishes or best interests; failing to provide agreed upon services to the elderly person (such as care giving, home or vehicle repairs, or financial management); using elderly person's credit cards for unauthorized purchases; using the elderly person's name to open new credit accounts; misusing the elderly person's Power of Attorney; changing the elderly person's Will, Trusts, or inheritance for the abuser's benefit, and out-and-out fraud by scams and/or schemes.

Elderly people comprise an increasingly large number of our population. Some reports indicate one of every seven Americans is a senior citizen, that is, over 60 years. Also, seniors are disproportionate victims in many scams and schemes. Some reasons for senior victimization may be:

- ☐ **Accessibility**. Retirement or physical restrictions make it probable they will be home.

- ☐ **Isolation.** Seniors may not have regular contact with relatives or friends. Con men prey on vulnerability and loneliness.

- ☐ **Money.** Seniors are targets because cons believe they have accumulated large sums of money over their lifetime.

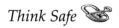

☐ **Declining Health**. Age, at some point, makes it difficult for many seniors to leave their homes, and it also impacts their ability to make home repairs.

Common Scams and Schemes

1. The Pigeon Drop

Several variations of the "pigeon drop" or "found money" scam exist. Common to all versions is that they claim a huge benefit for little investment. The event generally starts in a mall or shopping center environment. The target victim is approached by the con who engages the target with small talk to establish a friendly relationship. During the conversation, a second con approaches the two asking the target something like, "Did you drop this bag?" or, "Did you drop this envelope?" The cons then bait the target by opening the bag or envelope to find a large amount of cash. Of course, there is no identification with the money, which rules out returning the money to anyone.

The two cons get very excited about what they could each do with a share of the money, which sets up the target to believe that he/she will also get an equal share. At this point, greed generally overtakes intellect and the target is drawn in.

Recognizing the target has taken the bait, the cons suggest the found bag/envelope should be held for safekeeping for some period of time in case the owner is found. In the interim each should put up "good faith money." The cons convince the target that each put their good faith money into the bag/envelope and thus keep all the money together.

After the target has placed his/her money in the bag/envelope, the cons switch the container leaving the target with a similar container of like-weight, and the cons are off with the target's money.

For caregivers of elderly people – Banks and financial institutions may report to you if your elderly person attempts an unusual withdrawal, which may indicate they are involved in a scam. Talk with the institution about fraud alert.

2. Bank Examiner Fraud

Bank examiner fraud is not complicated. The con contacts a target, usually an elderly person, and poses as a police officer or bank official. The con puts emphasis on urgency and the need for the target to assist the bank in apprehending a teller who is stealing from customers. The target is asked to withdraw a large sum of money during which time investigators will be watching the transaction.

Upon leaving the bank, the withdrawal should be given to a waiting detective who will redeposit the money and complete the investigation. The con disappears with the money.

Again, banks and financial institutions may report to you, or some other responsible party, if your elderly person attempts an unusual withdrawal. These arrangements can be made through the financial institution.

3. Sweetheart Swindle

This scam has no gender limitations, and is successful because those targeted are often recently widowed, lonely, or depressed. These feelings make it easy for the con to befriend the target due to mental vulnerability. This scam is not limited to elderly people, however they often find themselves in situations that result in loneliness and depression, and are therefore an easier target.

The con capitalizes on the target's situation by telling the target everything he/she wants to hear. After gaining the target's trust, the con begins to siphon off money, jewelry, or any other asset they can get their hands on. The con lasts as long as it's beneficial, and then, most often, the criminal is off to another target. But sometimes these situations end in tragedy. Many cases have been documented where the con was able to get the target to make them the beneficiary of various assets, and the target was murdered as a result.

4. Home Repair

These cons go door-to-door offering a good cash deal on yard work, roof repairs, driveway repairs, etc. Often they claim the supplies were left over from another job thus the target can get a special deal. Once employed, one of two things may happen. One, the con says the job is larger than anticipated, and more time and materials are required. The con inflates the time and cost of materials and the target is billed up front an outrageous amount. The con gets the material money and is never seen again.

Or two, the con uses inferior products, does shoddy work or very little work at all. But the con always gets money upfront, and thus the homeowner has little recourse. These cons are unlicensed, have no roots, and simply disappear to another community.

5. Hiring a Contractor

Home repairs can be very expensive, and crooked contractors are abundant and eager to tell elderly homeowners exactly what they want to hear. They often promise things just short of miracles concerning their products and services to lure the elderly into the scam.

Avoidance is the best defense against these opportunistic contractors. Elderly people should not deal with an unlicensed contractor. Licensed contractors most generally need to pass a state administered test and/or have several years experience in the trade. Once licensed, the state can track complaints and the outcome of the complaint. These records are available to the general public and can most often be accessed by computer, free. Also, elderly people should check the workers' compensation policy to ensure workers are covered for any injury that might occur on the property.

Elderly people should take their time before making a decision about hiring a contractor, and get at least three bids and check with previous customers. And they shouldn't be shy about contacting previous customers. If they are happy with the work they often extend an invitation for other people to look at the job. They can also comment on timeliness of completion, cleanliness of the work environment, and meeting the budget, among others.

Elderly people should get a contract in writing, and review the contract with a trusted person prior to signing. The contract should include a specific description of work to be done, materials to be used, total cost of the project, and start and completion dates. They should also insist on a building permit (if required).

No one should ever pay cash for the job because it leaves no trail and you cannot put a stop payment on cash. Unfortunately, things don't always go well in contractor relationships. The ability to exercise some control, such as stop payment on a check, makes a good bargaining chip. Every contract should include a schedule of payments in writing, and people should resist pressure to paying ahead of time. Elderly people should keep extra funds available for additions or changes they may elect during the project.

Elderly people should remember to avoid door-to-door solicitations, and beware of high-pressure sales, demand for cash payments, and scare tactics such as faulty wiring or other emergencies as a result of a "free" inspection.

6. Telemarketing – Help is on the Way

Unscrupulous telemarketers are a serious threat to the unsuspecting; however, another aspect regarding telemarketers is almost as equally bad. That is, telemarketers who disrupt dinner or disturb rest or sleep. At least partial relief is available with the National Do-Not-Call List, which was established in 2003. People disturbed by certain telemarketing calls can silence these calls by registering for free in the Do-Not-Call program. These new federal rules, in part, require telemarketers to transmit identification information that can be viewed by a caller ID, and can limit hang ups or dead air on the line. But the relief is only partial because the National Registry does not stop every call. Only solicitations from certain businesses outside the consumer's home state are blocked, and charitable organizations are exempt. Other organizations exempt from the new rules include:

☐ Political groups;

☐ Businesses calling established customers;

☐ Banks, insurers and telephone companies.

Consumers can enroll through the Internet or a toll-free number and must renew registration every five years. Telemarketers must buy and check the list every three months to determine who does not want to be called. Serious penalties and fines may be imposed for each situation in which a listed person is called. Consumers will be able to file complaints by telephone or online to an automated system with the Federal Trade Commission (FTC).

The telephone is an instrument frequently used by fraudsters to take advantage of others because it can be so easy. All a criminal needs to run a telephone scam is a front. For example, to organize a phony charity, all you need is a fictitious charity and a list of telephone numbers. The best protection from these telephone scams is awareness.

7. Canadian Sweepstakes Scam

In this scam, the elderly are targeted because of their vulnerability. The ideal target is an elderly person living alone with infrequent contact with friends or relatives. Generally, the elderly person is contacted by telephone and told they have won a large amount of money in the Canadian (or other) Sweepstakes. However, in order to receive the money, they must first pay taxes on the winnings. Of course, there are no winnings and the fraud is most often completed when the fraudster receives the "so-called" tax money.

But sometimes they take it another step. On occasion, the fraudster will double-dip and ask for some other "fee" in connection with the winnings. The fraudster often diverts inquiry by representing himself or herself as a customs agent, Canadian investigator, or similar official. Similarly in domestic fraud, the person may represent himself or herself as a police officer or a federal agent.

8. Phony Vehicle Accident

Cons prey on the fact that many elderly view their driver's license as one of the last privileges of independence, therefore they tend to be very protective concerning anything that may jeopardize their license. In practicality, the scam is very simple. The cons, generally at least two are involved (one to claim damage and the other to claim to be a witness), target an elderly person entering a shopping center. In their absence, they put paint or another substance on the unattended vehicle. When the person returns to the vehicle, the cons suddenly appear and accuse the elderly person of hitting their vehicle and use the paint on their vehicle as evidence of damage. The cons then demand settlement for damages, or threaten to call the police. This is often enough to convince the elderly person to pay them off.

9. Distraction Burglary

Distraction burglary is a type of crime where a ruse rather than force is used to gain entry to steal. Common deception tactics include posing as a utility worker, police official, canvasser, or door-to-door sales person. Another favorite of distraction burglars is to use females with small children to contact the intended victim and keep their attention, while their cohort enters from another point. The intent is to distract and steal valuables of opportunity. The victims are usually females who live alone and are elderly. Defensive strategies should include:

☐ Put a peephole in the primary entrance door. Use it to identify callers.

☐ Put a chain-lock on the primary door, and put the chain in place before opening the door to strangers. But get in the habit of leaving it off for your fire safety.

☐ Visually examine the clothing of the caller. Does it seem to fit what the caller claims to be?

☐ Ask for an ID card, then close the door and check it out. Use the telephone book to get numbers; not a number supplied by the caller.

☐ If you are not completely satisfied, don't let them in. Notify the police.

☐ Don't admit strangers into your home.

10. Magazine Subscriptions

These cons use telephone sales pitches for free, pre-paid, or special magazine subscription deals. Salespeople encourage the elderly people to buy, but do not give total costs or offer magazines for just a few dollars a week. Often the elderly people pay hundreds of dollars over several years for subscriptions that sell elsewhere for less.

Use caution with door-to-door or telephone sales pitches for free, pre-paid, or special magazine subscription deals. Impulse purchases may leave you with monthly payments you may not want or could buy for less. And be particularly aware of multi-year subscriptions.

The Federal Trade Commission's Telemarketing Sales Rules require telemarketers to make certain disclosures and prohibits them from lying. It also requires the caller to cease calling if you ask to be put on the company's "do not call list." The FTC offers the following tips to deal with a telephone sales pitch for magazine subscriptions:

☐ The caller must promptly identify the seller and the purpose of the call. If the offer includes the promise of prizes or gifts, the sales pitch for the magazines must come first. If it doesn't, hang up. The caller is breaking the law.

☐ If you ordered magazines over the phone once, you may be called again. Although you may think the call is about customer satisfaction, chances are it's about renewals and additional subscriptions. Listen carefully to the offers to make sure you understand the terms.

☐ You may be called to renew your subscription, but the caller may not actually represent the publisher. Before you agree to renew, check the expiration date to determine how close it is. It's usually on the mailing label. Or, you may want to call the publisher to verify the expiration date and to confirm that the caller is authorized to renew your subscription.

☐ Ask for a written copy of the contract before you agree to buy any subscription. Read it. Make sure you understand what you'll get, the cost of each magazine and each subscription, and the cost of the entire package.

☐ Keep information about your bank accounts and credit cards to yourself – unless you know who you're dealing with. You may get a letter or postcard soliciting your business, or telling you that you've won a prize or contest. Often, this is a front for a scam. Instructions tell you to respond to a promoter with certain information. But if you give your bank account or credit card number over the phone to a stranger for "qualification," "verification" or, "computer purposes," it may be used to debit your account without your permission.

For Door-to-Door Magazine Sales the FTC offers the following tips:

☐ Beware of emotional appeals by someone selling door-to-door. For example, the student selling magazine subscriptions using the appeal that your sale will help him/her get a college scholarship or other such rewards.

☐ If you buy from a door-to-door salesperson in your home, and the purchase is more than $25, you're protected under the FTC's Cooling-Off Rule, which gives you three days to cancel your order and receive a full refund. The seller must inform you of your right to cancel, and give you a summary of your cancellation rights and two copies of the cancellation form.

☐ Ask to see the required cancellation notice before you agree to buy. If the salesperson doesn't have it, don't place an order. The company is breaking the law.

☐ For mailed postcards selling magazine subscriptions, the FTC offers the following tips:

✦ These postcards usually say nothing about magazine subscriptions, but direct you to call a telephone number about a contest, prize or sweepstakes entry.

✦ If you call, you may get information about prizes, gifts or other awards – but more than likely, you'll get a sales pitch for magazine subscriptions.

✦ According to the law, you never have to buy anything or pay to claim a prize, gift, or award.

✦ For phony magazine invoices or renewal notices, the FTC offers the following tips:

✦ These notices come in your mail and look like bills. If you already subscribe to the magazine, check the subscription expiration date.

✦ Also check the notice carefully to see if it came from the publisher.

✦ If you're not a subscriber and you didn't order any magazines, you're not obligated to pay.

The FTC works for consumers to prevent fraudulent, deceptive, and unfair business practices in the marketplace, and to provide information to help consumers spot, stop and avoid them. To file a complaint or to get information on consumer issues, visit www.ftc.gov or call toll-free, **1.877.FTC.HELP (1.877.382.4357): TTY: 1.866.653.4261.**

11. Credit and Charge Card Fraud/Theft

Credit and charge card fraud poses a double threat for the elderly. One threat is from a caregiver. Generally this caregiver is an adult child or spouse, may have a drug or alcohol abuse problem, and is dependent on the elderly person financially. The caregiver uses their position to gain control over the elderly person's finances, and then uses credit and charge cards for his/her personal needs.

The second threat is from theft, which can occur in several scenarios. For example, a thief goes through trash and finds discarded receipts or carbons, and then uses the account numbers. Or, a dishonest clerk makes an extra imprint from your credit or charge card, and uses it to make personal charges. Or

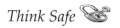

maybe the elderly person receives a letter or phone call with a message to call a number and claim a free prize. But first, they must join a club by supplying a credit card account number. This account number is then used for illegal purchases, and the prize never comes.

12. Caregiver Theft

The following behaviors may suggest caregivers are stealing from an elderly person:

- ☐ Caregiver asks only financial questions and does not ask questions related to eldercare;

- ☐ Caregiver has no obvious means of support;

- ☐ Problems with alcohol or drugs;

- ☐ Previous history of abuse;

- ☐ Anger or indifference toward the elder;

- ☐ Emotional or psychiatric problems;

- ☐ Inappropriate defensiveness;

- ☐ Aggressive toward elder;

- ☐ Exhibits concern that too much money is being spent on eldercare.

If you know or suspect an elderly person is being victimized, you must take action. Because an elderly victim is generally reluctant to report the abuse, a person's well-being may depend on you to recognize and report suspected abuse or theft.

Elderly People and Investment Fraud

Investment scams are not limited to elderly people. Following are investments all should be very cautious of:

1. Promissory Notes

Unlicensed brokers market many promissory notes. Elderly people should be aware of nine-month promissory notes in particular. These notes attempt to circumvent federal and state securities' laws; however, nine-month promissory notes are not exempt from regulatory controls. People should check with their state's investment and financing authority or the Securities Exchange Commission (SEC) for due diligence.

2. Internet Fraud

On-line trading has become a major issue in terms of trade execution, capacity, disclosure, margin, and suitability. A number of trading firms have given unlicensed investment advice, unlicensed broker-dealer activity, and fraud in connection with guaranteed results and promises of success.

3. Telemarketing Fraud

New high-pressure telephone sales operations open all the time, selling illegal and fraudulent investment products. Sales representatives will say anything to convince the investor to part with their money. They offer very high returns on investments, e.g., promissory notes with perhaps as much as a 12% monthly return.

Remember, risk and reward go hand-in-hand. If you are offered a high return with no risk, be very, very careful. Get the deal in writing, and ask a trusted financial person to evaluate it.

Elderly people should be cautious of any unknown person calling and soliciting funds. Be particularly careful if they involve:

- [ ] Free gifts that require payment of shipping and handling charges or other fees;

- [ ] Reluctance to provide written materials about the organization;

- [ ] Claims that you have won a prize that requires you to verify your credit card or checking account number;

- [ ] High-pressure pitches to "act now."

For example, in August of 2004 in Santa Clara County California, a con established an out-of-state front company alleging future sales would take off and create significant profits for partners. The con sold these partnerships for as much as $120,000 to elderly people as old as ninety-one, many of which he contacted through a senior center. At least forty-two people lost their money without hope of recovery, and the out-of-state company has since dissolved.

In September 2004, the *San Jose Mercury News* reported that over 135 people had been arrested during an investigation of global telemarketing scams. Five million victims, many of them elderly, had lost an estimated $1 billion in these scams. Among them, a $500 million phone billing scam that included a fake call center where bogus operators tried to talk customers into paying fictitious charges. The investigation also uncovered bogus lottery and sweepstakes scams, fake pre-approved credit cards, offers of non-existent investments, tax evasion scams, and people posing as law enforcement officers to recoup fictitious charges.

4. Viatical Investments

Viatical investment companies solicit investors to buy interests in the death benefits provided in life insurance policies of terminally ill patients. The insured receives a discounted percentage of the death benefits in cash to allegedly improve the quality of their lives in the final days. These investments must be considered extremely speculative and are only appropriate for persons willing to risk losing all their investment.

5. Entertainment Scams

Many scams offer opportunities for investments in movie deals and other entertainment products with promises of guaranteed profits without disclosing the risk. This is another scam that uses the telephone. The caller represents that he/she is part of an investment group putting together a major film deal. The film star is a major (unnamed) player in the industry, and the offer is a ground floor opportunity to make lots of money. No risk is mentioned, and the caller claims it to be a once in a lifetime investment opportunity. However, your decision must be made immediately. Remember:

☐ Get the deal in writing before investing.

☐ Urgency is a tip-off to a scam.

☐ Review the deal with a trusted financial person.

In these situations, probably no such film exists, and if there is, it is not likely to be a moneymaker. So think about it; with all the "money professionals" in the film industry, why would it be necessary for this caller to look outside the industry for small investor funding?

6. Ponzi/Pyramid Schemes

A pyramid scheme involves the collection of money from individuals at the bottom (new investors) to pay initial investors at the top, with all the emphasis on bringing in new members and not on selling the product or service. In these scams, the newest members/investors lose all their money.

One tactic fraudsters often use to lure a potential target is the bait of "Minor Investment – Tremendous Returns." That's the essence of the pyramid scheme. The idea is that you send an agreed upon sum of money to invest in the program. An administrator distributes those monies to prior members, and puts your name at the bottom of the list. As new members join, their sum is distributed upward, and you get a share of that sum. You are sold on the idea that the number of people below you will grow and you will share in vast profit. But the following problems exist:

☐ ALL Pyramid schemes are illegal.

☐ The sum of money put in the scheme never appreciates. It is merely redistributed less fees taken by the administrator.

☐ Mathematically, at some point, not enough new members join to support the distributions and the scheme collapses (US Securities and Exchange Commission).

☐ The only money made in these schemes by some people (initial members) is at the expense of subsequent members.

Several variations to the scheme exist, but common to all is the use of new recruit money to pay off early investors.

Avoid Investment Fraud

Unscrupulous stockbrokers and financial planners who engage in abusive practices often seek out the elderly, according to the California Department of Corporations, the California regulator of firms and individuals in the securities and investment industry. A critical step in wise investing for any individual is taking the time to check backgrounds of potential brokers and advisors prior to entering into financial relationships. Individual investors can check with the Securities Exchange Commission (SEC) for information on a financial advisor.

Additionally, investors may avoid mistakes by using the following tips:

☐ Don't be a courtesy victim. Con artists don't hesitate to take advantage of people using good manners. A stranger who calls either on the telephone or at your door should be regarded with utmost caution.

☐ Say NO to anyone who presses you into an immediate decision, particularly if they don't provide an opportunity to check out the salesperson or firm.

☐ Stay in charge of your money. Be aware of any professional who suggests putting your money into something you don't understand, or who promises to "take care of everything for you." Constant vigilance is a necessary part of being a successful investor.

☐ Never judge a person's integrity by how they sound. Successful con artists sound extremely professional and combine professional sounding sales pitches with extremely polite manners. Don't be fooled. Good manners and a slick sales pitch have nothing to do with real integrity, and have no bearing on the soundness of an investment opportunity.

☐ Watch out for salespeople who prey on your fears. Con artists take advantage of elderly people who fear that they will outlive their savings, or that all their financial resources will disappear as a result of a catastrophe. Fear and greed can cloud good judgment to the detriment of sound financial decisions. If the investment doesn't make sense, or if it seems too good to be true, it may be a scam.

☐ Older women with little investment experience should exercise particular caution. A con artist's ideal victim is the elderly widow. Elderly women on their own with little investment experience should always seek the advice of family members or a disinterested professional before deciding what to do with their savings.

☐ Monitor your investments. Many elderly people who trust unscrupulous investment people to make financial decisions compound the error by failing to keep an eye on the progress of the investment. Insist on regular written and oral reports.

☐ Look for trouble if retrieving your principle or cashing out profits is difficult. A stockbroker or other investment advisor who fails to respond to a request for a refund of the initial principle or profit from an investment may be a con artist. Unscrupulous investment professionals pocket the funds, and often go to great lengths in explaining why investments or profits are not readily accessible. If the investment is not a fixed term, such as a bond, a request for a refund of principle or profits should be available to the investor within a reasonable amount of time.

☐ Don't let embarrassment or fear keep you from reporting investment fraud. Con artists recognize the fears of many elderly people and count on these fears to keep them in business.

☐ Beware of "relate" scams. Elderly people who possess a finite amount of money, which is unlikely to be replenished in the event of fraud will sometimes go along with another scheme, if faced with a loss of funds. These so-called "second bite" scams defraud investors who have already been victimized. Be very suspicious of promises to "make good" on original funds that were lost, with an even greater return than was originally promised.

Credit/Charge Card Fraud Prevention Strategies (Also See Identify Theft)

Several strategies are helpful to guarding yourself against credit card fraud. Things to do:

☐ Sign your credit cards as soon as they arrive.

☐ Carry your cards separately from your wallet, in a zippered compartment, a business card holder, or another small pouch.

☐ Keep a record of account numbers, their expiration dates, and the phone number and address of each company in a secure place.

☐ Keep an eye on your card during a transaction, and get it back as quickly as possible. Confirm that it is your card.

☐ Destroy carbons.

☐ Save receipts to compare with billing statements.

- [ ] Open bills promptly and reconcile accounts monthly.
- [ ] Report any questionable charges promptly and in writing to the card issuer.
- [ ] Notify card companies in advance of a change of address.
- [ ] Shred all documents that contain personal information.

DO NOT:

- [ ] Lend your credit/charge card to anyone.
- [ ] Leave cards or receipts lying around.
- [ ] Sign a blank receipt.
- [ ] Write your account number on a postcard or the outside of an envelope.
- [ ] Give out your account number over the phone unless you're making the call to a company you know is reputable.

Warning Signs of Financial Exploitation

As people age, they often become more dependent and may need help with many of the tasks of daily living. Some lose functional capacity and become vulnerable to financial exploitation.

Signs of exploitation may be:

- [ ] Unusual activity in bank accounts, such as withdrawal from ATM when the elder cannot walk or get to the bank.
- [ ] Signatures on checks and other documents that do not resemble the elderly person's signature.
- [ ] Checks and other documents are signed when the elderly person cannot write.
- [ ] Lack of amenities such as TV, grooming items, appropriate clothing.
- [ ] Changes in spending patterns. The elderly person buys things they do not have a need for.

☐ Numerous unpaid bills and overdue rent when someone is designated to pay bills.

☐ The elderly person has been placed in a nursing home or residential care facility that is inconsistent with their income or assets.

☐ The person controlling the elderly person's resources denies the elderly person necessary placement and/or services. The controller won't spend money because they want to preserve potential inheritance.

Strategies for Elderly People to Protect their Finances:

☐ DO NOT let anyone threaten or intimidate you. If someone close to you is trying to take control of your finances, speak to someone you TRUST or call a protective service organization.

☐ Plan ahead to protect your assets to ensure that your wishes are followed. Talk to someone at your bank, an attorney, or financial advisor about the best options for you.

☐ Check references and credentials of anyone who wants to do work in your home.

☐ DO NOT allow employees access to or information pertaining to your finances.

☐ Get to know your banker. Build a relationship with the people who handle your finances. They can look for suspicious activity related to your account.

☐ Consult with a financial advisor or attorney before signing any document.

☐ NEVER allow someone to rush you into a deal. Ask for details in writing.

☐ Pay with checks and credit cards rather than cash to keep a paper trail.

☐ Stay informed about current scams and con games. AARP is a good source of information (www.AARP.org).

☐ DO NOT feel afraid to say "NO."

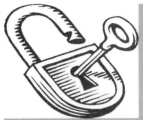

Section Four – Safety Precautions at Work

- CHAPTER 12 - WORKPLACE VIOLENCE
- CHAPTER 13 - SEXUAL HARASSMENT

Introduction

Managers and business leaders hold many responsibilities in an organization. But perhaps the most difficult task they must perform is to oversee the well-being of all their employees. Depending on the size of the organization, this may involve anywhere from two to one hundred people. In smaller organizations, spotting and addressing problems in troubled employees before they affect their work performance is easy. You can tell when something is wrong when you're only in charge of a few people. But if you're in charge of a hundred people, you may have trouble remembering their names, let alone determining whether they're having a bad day.

With such a huge workforce to oversee, you may not notice destructive patterns unless they start to affect work performance. Unfortunately, at that point, it may be too late. So what can a manager of a huge number of people do to keep the workplace safe? The key to safety is always awareness. When managers are aware that workplace violence is a nationwide problem, they know what to look for in their current employees, they know how to identify violent potential in new employees, and they know how to deal with problems as they arise. Only then can they increase the level of safety in their organization. The following chapters will give managers and business leaders the traits, behaviors, and patterns to stop before a violent outburst happens.

Chapter 12   WORKPLACE VIOLENCE

W orkplace violence committed by employees or former employees is one of the fastest growing problems in Corporate America. According to the FBI report, Workplace Violence: Issues in Response, March 2004, there were seven co-workers killed by a technician in Hawaii in 1999, seven slain by a software engineer in Massachusetts in 2000, four killed by a former forklift driver in Chicago in 2001, three killed by an insurance executive in New York City in 2002, three killed by a plant worker in Missouri in 2003, and six killed by a plant worker in Mississippi in 2003.

These issues receive sensational press coverage because of the degree of violence; however, they do not represent the typical incidents that managers or employees encounter in the workplace.

Category of violent victimization in the workplace	Percent reported to the police
Rape/sexual assault	23.6%
Robbery	71.4
Aggravated assault	64.3
Simple assault	41.1

Occupational field	Crime reported to police
Medical	39.6%
Mental health	22.9
Teaching	28.1
Law enforcement	74.8
Retail sales	53.9
Transportation	37.0
Other	38.7

Workplace Violence: A Report to the Nation, University of Iowa Injury Prevention Research Center. Iowa City, Iowa: Feburary 2001: Violence in the Workplace 1993-1999 Special Report, U.S. Department of Justice. Office of Justice Programs, Bureau of Justice Statistics Washington D.C.: December 2001. NCJ 190076

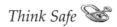

But few companies are prepared to handle any type of violent incident or threat in their organizations. However, organizations can do two things to reduce the probability of violent episodes:

+ **Number One:** Pre-employment background checks and drug screening. After all, the best deterrent to workplace violence is not to hire potentially troublesome or aggressive people in the first place. Hiring practices that check records (criminal, employment, driving, etc.) and that investigate contradictory information will help keep problem people out of the workplace.

+ **Number Two:** Organizations must confront the potential for workplace violence with programs that demonstrate to employees that threats or intimidation – even in jest – will not be tolerated, and severe consequences for minor infractions can be expected. Some actions a proactive company may take include:

  ☐ Establish a no tolerance policy concerning threats, intimidation and violence. All employees should read, sign, and get a copy of the policy.

  ☐ Establish procedures for dealing with threats and threat behavior.

  ☐ Establish a trained incident response team with access to threat assessment professionals.

  ☐ Set consistent, effective disciplinary procedures.

Warning Signs of Potentially Violent Individuals

No precise method for predicting an episode of violence exists. But a person may display one or more of the following warning signs before becoming violent. Realize, though, these signs do NOT necessarily indicate that an individual WILL become violent. A display of the following signs should trigger concern, as people experiencing problems usually exhibit one or more of them:

☐ Irrational beliefs and ideas;

☐ Verbal, nonverbal or written threats or intimidation;

☐ Fascination with weaponry and/or acts of violence;

☐ Expressions of a plan to hurt himself or others;

☐ Externalization of blame;

☐ Unreciprocated romantic obsession;

☐ Taking up large amounts of a supervisor's time with behavior or performance problems;

☐ Eliciting a fear reaction from co-workers/clients (a "bully" personality). This person may also be feared because of his/her size, language or intimidating action such as shadow boxing or striking objects

☐ Drastic change in belief systems;

☐ Displays of unwarranted anger;

☐ New or increased level of stress at home or work;

☐ Inability to take criticism;

☐ Feelings of being victimized;

☐ Intoxication from alcohol or other substances at work;

☐ Expressions of hopelessness or heightened anxiety;

☐ Productivity and/or attendance problems;

☐ Violence towards inanimate objects;

☐ Steals or sabotages projects or equipment;

☐ Lack of concern for the safety of others.

Recognizing Inappropriate Behavior

Inappropriate behavior is often a warning sign of potential hostility or violence, and when left unchecked it can escalate to higher levels. Co-workers who exhibit the following behaviors should be reported to a manager and Human Resources, if one exists in the company:

☐ Unwelcome name-calling, obscene language, or other abusive behavior;

☐ Intimidation through direct or veiled verbal threats;

☐ Throwing objects in the workplace regardless of the size, the type of object being thrown, or whether a person is the target of a thrown object;

☐ Physically touching another employee in an intimidating, malicious, or sexually harassing manner (including hitting, slapping, poking, kicking, pinching, grabbing, and pushing);

☐ Physically intimidating others (including obscene gestures, getting in someone's face, and fist shaking).

High Risk Behavior to Watch For

The following behaviors identify a very troubled co-worker who may be moving from a potential violent risk toward acting out a violent episode.

1. Change of Behavior

Human beings are creatures of habit. People repeat behaviors such as waking for work, showering, drying their hair, and leaving for work at the same time, or at least within minutes of the same time, day after day. Other patterns also follow day after day such as early arrival at work and going to the cafeteria to socialize over morning coffee with fellow workers or arrival at work early to line up work for the day. With a troubled employee, some changes are obvious, while others are subtle. But their normal patterns will certainly be interrupted. Apparent changes may include an increasing lack of interest in group activities, breaking social contacts, or no longer talking about themselves or their personal activities. A subtle change could be someone who used to smile frequently, and now forces emotions.

A troubled co-worker often has a strong desire to be away from others. They keep a high degree of secretiveness in their lives, and when they do interact with others, it is generally brief and concise. They have poor social skills and tend to keep their private lives extremely private. Troubled people do not party or socialize with other employees during lunch or break periods.

2. Threats

Threats may be overt or covert. Overt threats frequently come from disgruntled and angry co-workers. You may notice a sense of getting even demonstrated in their attitude. They may also be openly hostile or have an explosive temper. They tend to blame others for mistakes, and they make comments such as, "If I get fired, I'm coming back to get even," or, "I should shoot the supervisor."

Covert threats may be more difficult to detect. Open hostility may not be present; however, the person fosters a desire to get back at or even with someone in the workplace. No specific statements for harm exist, but statements like, "I'm fed up with this," or, "I can't take this anymore," are likely.

Another aspect of threat is intimidation, which may take the form of attitude, language, or eye contact. Being around this type of person creates a very uncomfortable and undesirable feeling.

3. Mood Swings

Mood swings can be described as happy at one point, then depressed the next, and could be as frequent as an hour or two apart. They may be the result of work related issues, non-work related issues, or both. When anticipating contact with this type of person, you never know what to expect.

Strategies to De-escalate Potentially Violent Situations

Unpleasant human interactions occur at, and away from, work on a regular basis. The following suggestions focus on things to avoid during such encounters. These suggestions are intended to de-escalate the situation and prevent violence. But if at any time a person's behavior starts to escalate toward violence, disengage. Trained professionals should be brought in to deal with violent people.

Things to DO and NOT DO:

☐ DO NOT speak in a patronizing or run around manner.
   DO listen carefully and project calmness.

☐ DO NOT reject demands initially.
   DO listen with empathy.

☐ DO NOT position body in an aggressive manner such as directly in front of with hands on hips.
   DO stand at right angles with relaxed and attentive posture.

☐ DO NOT make sudden moves.
   DO speak softly and non-threatening.

☐ DO NOT threaten or belittle.
   DO acknowledge the person's feelings and acknowledge they are upset.

Think Safe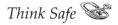

☐ DO NOT criticize the agitated person.
  <u>DO</u> give the person time to calm down.

☐ DO NOT make the situation seem less serious.
  <u>DO</u> be reassuring and point out choices.

☐ DO NOT take sides or agree with distortions.
  <u>DO</u> accept criticism in a positive way.

This is not a comprehensive list of techniques for reducing anger in others. But it sufficiently demonstrates that to respond with aggressive actions will only solicit an aggressive response.

Chapter 13

SEXUAL HARASSMENT

E veryone has a right to feel safe and secure at work or at school. Unwelcome sexual advances, requests for sexual favors, and other verbal or physical conduct of a sexual nature are not only unacceptable behavior, but in many instances they are also unlawful.

A precise legal definition of sexual harassment is difficult because of the continuing evolution and interpretation by the courts. Simply put, harassment can be verbal or physical, and it must be unwanted, protested, and continued, but is not necessarily sexual in nature. However, it must inhibit a person's work or affect productivity.

Both state and federal authorities generally cover laws relative to sexual harassment in the workplace. The federal agency responsible for handling sexual harassment complaints is the Equal Employment Opportunity Commission (EEOC). The EEOC has defined two areas that establish criteria for legal action:

☐ Quid pro quo sexual harassment

☐ Hostile environment sexual harassment

Quid Pro Quo Sexual Harassment

Quid pro quo sexual harassment is related to sexual advances or conduct of a sexual nature in exchange for continued employment, promotion, grades, or teaching advantage. The harassment can occur in a variety of circumstances, including, but not limited to, the following:

☐ The victim, as well as the harasser, may be a woman or man. The victim does not have to be of the opposite sex.

☐ The harasser can be the victim's supervisor, an agent of the employer, a supervisor in another area, a co-worker, a non-employee, or instructor.

☐ The victim does not have to be the person harassed but could be anyone affected by the offensive conduct.

☐ Unlawful sexual harassment may occur without economic injury to or discharge of the victim.

☐ The harasser's conduct must be unwelcome.

From an investigative point of view, the victim must ask the harasser to stop the unwelcome behavior. This communication must be professional and absent of humor or misinterpretation of message. The victim should also advise the Human Relations Department, chancellor's office, or whatever complaint resolution process is available in their particular organization.

Hostile Environment Sexual Harassment

Hostile environment sexual harassment occurs when the workplace culture commonly includes offensive or intimidating language, sexual comments or innuendo, pictures, touching, or request for sexual relations. Again, the activity must interfere with job performance, or create a hostile, intimidating, or offensive work environment. In these cases, an employer may be liable if:

☐ The employer knew or should have known about the harassment,

and

☐ The employer failed to take appropriate corrective action.

An employer may also be liable for a hostile environment created by others such as customers or independent contractors, provided the employer is aware of the harassment and fails to act. Knowledge may be established by:

☐ A complaint;

☐ No established policies against harassment;

☐ Harassment is open or widespread.

Remember, everyone has a right to feel safe and secure in the workplace. Ignoring sexual harassment will not make it go away. In fact, to refrain from addressing the issue may encourage the harasser because the whole point of the harassment is over control.

Strategies for consideration if you believe you are being harassed

- ☐ The EEOC requires all employers with more than 15 employees to have policies and procedures to address sexual harassment. Get a copy of this document and review it for application in your case.

- ☐ **Speak out timely.** Recognize that you are the victim. An annoyance or uncomfortable feeling may be the first indication of harassment. Trust your feelings and speak out clearly and definitively to your human relations department. This may be a formal or informal complaint.

- ☐ **Use caution**. Process is important to ensure that you do not become involved in a character defamation suit. Follow company or school policies and procedures.

- ☐ **Substantiate.** Record in writing all events of harassment in detail. Answer the questions: who, what, where, why, when and how. Don't forget to record name or names of witnesses.

- ☐ **Internal Assistance.** Internal resources are often the best place to start because the law clearly puts the company or school on notice that they must ensure a hassle-free environment. Thus companies/schools have a vested interest in getting the situation resolved.

- ☐ **External Assistance.** Seek an attorney who specializes in employment discrimination for advice. The attorney will be knowledgeable about statutes, filing dates, etc.

Section Five – Consumer Fraud Prevention

- CHAPTER 14 - CONSUMER FRAUD
- CHAPTER 15 - IDENTITY THEFT

Introduction

Throughout history, some people have always tried their best to take advantage of their fellow man to get their money. Unfortunately, no end to this phenomenon is in sight, and the list of ways and methods for scamming people out of their money have increased exponentially. But when people are aware of existing scams, and the potential for them to occur, they have a lower chance for falling victim. As scammers get smarter and more difficult to detect, potential victims must also increase their awareness. Perhaps the most important point to keep in mind is that you must question everything, especially when it sounds too good to be true.

Many of these scams are also covered in chapter eleven for elderly people, but they are so prevalent, the message is worth repeating for a general audience. The following chapters will make you aware of some existing scams, and provide you with insight into the mindset of the scammer. Therefore, as they become better, hopefully you'll be equipped with the knowledge of where and how they tend to strike.

Chapter 14 | CONSUMER FRAUD

Fraud is defined as an intentional perversion of truth to induce another person to part with something of value or to surrender a legal right. This definition has been simplified over the years into proverbs like: "There's no such thing as a free lunch," "There's a sucker born every minute," and, "Keep your eye on the donut and not on the hole." In fact, truth is embedded in these words. Following are examples that tend to prove the aforementioned proverbs are words of wisdom.

Magazine Subscription Scams

Remember, telephone sales pitches for free, pre-paid, or special magazine subscription deals should be examined very carefully. A spur of the moment purchase could result in several years of monthly payments of magazines that you may not want, or that you could buy for less. Additionally, you may be legally obligated to pay for a subscription you verbally agree to.

Keep the following tips in mind when you get a telephone solicitation for magazines:

☐ The solicitor must promptly identify the purpose of the call. If gifts or prizes are involved, the sales pitch for magazines must come first. If it doesn't, the solicitor is breaking the law, and you should break off the call.

☐ Once you've ordered magazines by phone, you are likely to get subsequent calls that lead you to believe it's a customer service call. However, it's about renewals or additional subscriptions. Listen carefully and understand exactly what the call is about.

☐ Always check your expiration date before renewing a subscription. Often they ask for a renewal with months still left on your

121

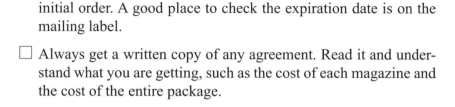

initial order. A good place to check the expiration date is on the mailing label.

☐ Always get a written copy of any agreement. Read it and understand what you are getting, such as the cost of each magazine and the cost of the entire package.

Door-to-door sales are another risky way to buy, and often magazine salespeople use this method of home contact. If you buy from a door-to-door salesperson and the purchase exceeds $25, you have three days to cancel the order without penalty. The salesperson must advise you of this and provide two copies of a cancellation notice.

The Federal Trade Commission works for the consumer to prevent fraudulent, deceptive, and unfair business practices in the marketplace, and to provide information to help consumers spot, stop, and avoid them. To file a complaint or get free information on consumer issues call toll free – **1.877.383.4357** or go to their web site at www.ftc.gov.

Telemarketing Travel Fraud

Telemarketing travel scams often begin with a potential target victim filling out an information card at a county fair, restaurant, or similar place. A follow-up telemarketing call is then made to the target consumer to tell them they have won an opportunity for a bargain vacation. But the bargain vacation is likely encumbered with hidden charges, such as mandatory upgrades, room fees, port charges, and service fees. Additionally, after you pay these "fees," restrictive travel dates may prohibit you from ever getting to use the trip at all.

Telemarketing sales pitches usually include:

☐ **Misrepresentations.** Pitches in these scams vary, but always offer a "deal." The deal is impossible to deliver, but you won't find out until your money has been extracted.

☐ **High pressure**. The caller may say you must buy right now or lose the opportunity. Any "deal" that requires an immediate response or you lose out probably isn't that great a deal. Back off and reconsider what you're getting into.

Don't become a victim. Consider the following:

☐ Be cautious of super deals, because businesses always operate to make a profit. Legitimate businesses are unlikely to offer deep discounts or give away products.

☐ Resist making snap decisions. Legitimate businesses do not exist on pressure tactics.

☐ Get details on exactly what you are paying for, especially with travel deals. Get the itinerary with specifics on all transportation and appurtenant arrangements. Determine what happens if you must cancel.

☐ Get everything you agree to in writing before you pay.

☐ Do not use debit or credit cards with anyone you don't know or haven't done business with previously over the telephone. Instead, pay by credit card on an invoice, and do not send cash.

☐ Paying by credit card has a couple advantages: one, you may have legal remedy for fraudulent charges; and two, you can dispute charges with your credit card issuer and perhaps have the charges reversed.

☐ Check with consumer protection agencies in your local government or get free information from Federal Trade Commission at **1.877.383.4357** or visit www.ftc.gov.

Bank Debit and Charge Cards

Automatic debit is simply an electronic withdrawal from your checking account, which offers a convenient method to pay obligations. However, if unprotected, electronic cards may also become a convenient method to steal your money.

Fraudulent telemarketers are highly skilled at getting unsuspecting victims to reveal financial information. They use promises of special deals, prizes, trips, awards, and anything else that may appeal to a vulnerable person. Most often these promises sound too good to be true. But at some point in the conversation, the fraudulent telemarketer will make a move to get a debit card number, a bank charge number, or a checking account number.

Frequently the telemarketer attempts to get your checking account number because with it, they can put a "demand draft" on your account. A demand draft does not require a signature, and automatically transfers the draft amount to the telemarketer's bank.

Remember, when you give anyone your bankcard number or checking account number, you have provided an opportunity for that person to access and withdraw money from your accounts.

Sweepstakes Fraud

Sweepstakes fraud usually begins with a mail or telephone contact that offers a valuable prize or award (the bait). The prize or award depends upon a contribution to a bogus charity, or buying some overpriced product or service. In this scam, "winners" almost always have to pay to play. However, skill contests are an exception to the pay-to-play scam.

Skill contests are won based on skill, knowledge, or talent. These lack the element of chance and may legally require entrants to buy something, make a payment, or a donation. Predators take advantage of the legality of skill contests to lure victims into their scheme by using simple initial issues. After the victim has taken the bait, the questions get more difficult and the fees continue to increase. Rarely, does the victim win anything in the end.

Don't become a victim. Remember:

☐ Legitimate contests do not require you to pay anything.

☐ Bulk mail "winners" are highly unlikely.

☐ Never speed mail checks or money orders, because then the thieves get your money more quickly. And think about what you are doing.

☐ Don't be tricked by mail that looks like, but is not really from, a well-known organization.

☐ Never disclose your credit card, debit, or checking account numbers.

☐ Marketers sell information gathered from various sources. Be careful when disclosing personal information for contests. You may get on a list you don't want to be on.

☐ Read everything carefully.

☐ Resist impulsive actions.

Charitable Donations

Fundraisers are either professional paid staff or volunteers of an organization. Professional fundraisers keep a portion of the collected revenue agreed to with the charity. Sometimes they retain a higher percentage than the charity actually receives, and other times they only keep a fraction of each contribution. Before contributing to any charity, you may want to ask how much of your money actually goes toward the cause. But the decision whether to donate is best made on a case-by-case basis. If you think the retention is too high, seek other options for giving. Asking how your contribution will be distributed is always a good idea.

Tax-Exempt vs. Tax-Deductible

Many times contributors confuse the terms tax-exempt and tax-deductible, and agree to a donation expecting a write-off. Tax-exempt means the organization does not have to pay taxes. But tax-deductible means a contribution may be deducted on your federal income tax return. Just because an organization is tax-exempt does not mean the contribution is tax-deductible. The distinction is important because unethical organizations will represent themselves as a tax-deductible charity when in fact they are a tax-exempt organization. This deception could cost you a deduction.

Other variations of this confusion come from words on receipts such as "important, keep this receipt for future reference," or similar statements which imply the contribution is tax deductible. Actually, these words do not have any relevance at all to the issue of taxation.

Predators may also invent fictitious charities and keep all the money. After a period, they close shop on that fictitious charity and invent another. Frequently, they call on previous contributors, and thus continue a cycle of fraud.

Charities play a significant role in helping the sick and needy, and most use contributions prudently. However, others may spend an inordinate amount on fundraising and administrative expenses. Remember, before you give to an unknown charity or group, check them out through the Better Business Bureau, or try www.give.org.

Fraudulent Loan Brokers

When money is involved, someone will always try to make a fast buck by fraud. This certainly is true in the money lending business. Fraudulent loan brokers and other individuals offering credit services are not difficult to find. A favorite scam used by these people is the advance fee loan. Advance fee purports you get a guaranteed loan or other credit; however, you must pay a fee before you apply.

In this scam, the predator advertises in media outlets likely to reach people with no credit, bad credit, or bankruptcy. Ads may appear in mailers, community newsletters, or tacked on utility poles or vacant structures. The advertisement suggests, or may even guarantee, a loan despite previous credit difficulties. Additionally, the advertisement lists a telephone number for contact, but intentionally avoids a physical address. The predator extracts as large a fee as possible from the unsuspecting victim, who believes their loan is inevitable. The predator then takes the fee and disappears. But the victim has little recourse because the predator does not leave a trail.

To protect yourself from these scams, avoid the following situations:

- ☐ It's against the law for anyone to ask you to pay, or for them to accept payment, for his or her service until you get the loan or credit. If you don't have the approval paperwork in hand when asked to pay, don't.

- ☐ Be cautious in any business deal of a company that has no physical address. It does not mean that a company is not legitimate, but without a physical address complaints may be difficult to resolve. Without a location, you are at the mercy of someone returning a phone call. Then the legal process becomes difficult, and an additional expense to locate the company is probable.

Credit Card Protection Scam

In most, if not all cases, liability for unauthorized charges to credit card is limited to fifty dollars. Because of consumer uncertainty, predators have found an opportunity to take advantage and fleece the public with so-called credit card loss protection insurance. This approach convinces the consumer that they are liable for all unauthorized charges. Their methods vary, but all attempt to instill fear of loss of your hard earned money. Some examples:

- ☐ The caller is from the issuing institution's security department and wants to update their protection.

- ☐ The law has changed and you are now responsible for all unauthorized charges.

- ☐ Computer hackers can take over your account and max out your card.

These callers scam believers into buying essentially worthless protection. Consumers are not actually responsible for unauthorized charges over fifty dollars. Consumers, however, must follow the issuer's procedure for notification and dispute of unauthorized charges to be covered with this provision.

The following is worth repeating: **NEVER** give out personal information unless you have initiated a telephone call and know whom you are talking to. Scammers will use your personal information, or sell it to others, to commit fraud, theft, or both. With your personal information, the thief may establish credit in your name and charge substantial amounts to you.

Investment Fraud

Most everyone has received the seductive Nigerian Letter that has secreted government funds that can only be released by the recipient sending an appropriate sum of money. Supposedly, this money allows the release of said government money with the promise of vast returns.

The film production scam offer is another popular one, which offers opportunity to invest in a high-quality, low budget family film with actors who sacrifice high salaries and thus "guarantee" a high return on the investment. The money invested supposedly goes to production, distribution, and screenplay development. And several other popular methods exist, such as oil company scams and rare coin scams. Obviously in the foregoing, the Nigerian Letter is out-and-out fraud. No such government funds exist. The film scammers get all the money because they are the producers and screenwriters. Oil field surveys are also false, and rare coins are marked up so high there rarely is a profit.

Predators can easily make investment scams seem very exciting, almost like absolute moneymakers. Often they establish elaborate fronts with office space and vehicles to camouflage their fraudulent investment pitch. However it seems that the extra efforts are not always necessary, because the Nigerian Letter has been around for years. And some even fall prey to it. Recently, an administrative assistant embezzled a very large sum of money from her employer to invest in this scam. She stated she intended to put the embezzled funds back from the millions she gained from her venture. However, she realized she was cheated out of the money when she lost all contact with the promoter.

Everyone is a potential target for predators primarily because they are smooth, articulate, and experts at taking advantage. But fraud is always a possibility in any investment. So before making any investment, research the opportunity, contact the Better Business Bureau, understand the risk, and beware of offers that sound too good to be true. One last word, sure things don't exist.

Reduce Exposure to Fraud

Everyone, at one time or the other, has been inundated with unsolicited mail, telemarketing, and/or email. Fortunately, the opportunity to reduce these mailings, calls, and emails now exists. Start with the three major credit bureaus. By notifying the credit bureaus that you do not want your personal information shared for promotional purposes, you can eliminate unsolicited mail. Correspondence for the major credit bureaus should be directed to the following addresses:

Trans Union, Marketing List Opt Out
PO Box 97328
Jackson, MS 39288-7388
(www.transunion.com)

Experian, Consumer Opt-Out
701 Experian Parkway
Allen, TX 75013
(www.experian.com)

Equifax, Inc. Options
PO Box 740123
Atlanta, GA 30374-0123
(www.equifax.com)

To remove your name from marketing lists, credit bureaus offer an "Opt-Out" option. Call toll-free at **1.888.567.8688**. Also, the Direct Marketing Association (DMA) offers mail and telephone preference services that allow you to reduce the amount of direct mail marketing and telemarketing you receive. When you register, your name will be put on a delete file. Following are the addresses:

DMA Mail Preference Service
PO Box 9008
Farmingdale, NY 11735-9008

DMA Telephone Preference Service
PO Box 9014
Farmingdale, NY 11735-9014

Additionally, you can opt-out of unsolicited commercial email through the DMA Email Preference Service. Contact DMA at www.e-mps.org.

Chapter 15

IDENTITY THEFT

Identity theft involves acquiring key pieces of someone's identifying personal information, such as bank and credit card numbers, income level, social security number, name, mother's maiden name, address, and phone number, and then pretending to be that person. Commonly, an identity thief uses personal information to open a credit card account or for numerous other financial crimes.

Thieves use a number of ways to gain access to your personal data. Some of the ways include:

- ☐ They steal wallets or purses containing credit and bankcards, and identification.

- ☐ They steal mail that includes bank and credit card statements, pre-approved credit offers, calling cards, etc.

- ☐ They search through garbage at homes and businesses for personal data. This act is commonly referred to as dumpster diving.

- ☐ They divert mail from your home by submitting a change of address form.

- ☐ They use personal information you share on the Internet.

- ☐ They work with insiders at banks, department stores, etc. to get personal information.

After acquiring these personal identifiers, the thief can then take over your identity. Thieves use the personal information to:

- ☐ Telephone your credit card issuer and pretend to be you. They request a mailing address change for the credit card account. The account is run up, and because the bills are going to a new address, it may take an extended period of time before the crime is uncovered.

☐ Open a new credit card account using your name, date of birth, and social security number. When they don't pay the bills, the delinquent account is reported to a credit agency.

☐ Establish phone or wireless service in your name.

☐ Use counterfeit checks or debit cards and drain your bank account.

☐ Buy cars by taking out auto loans in your name.

By managing personal information, with an awareness of the problem, certain strategies may reduce or minimize risk.

These strategies are as follows:

☐ Promptly remove mail from the mailbox after delivery.

☐ Deposit outgoing mail in Post Office collection mailboxes. Do not leave it in unsecured mail receptacles.

☐ Never give personal information over the telephone unless you initiated the phone call. Protect this information and release it only when absolutely necessary.

☐ Shred pre-approved credit applications, credit card reports, bills, and other financial information before discarding.

☐ Empty your wallet of extra credit cards and IDs, and cancel the ones you don't use. Maintain a list of the ones you keep.

☐ Order your credit report from the three credit bureaus once a year to check for fraudulent activity or other discrepancies.

☐ Never leave receipts at bank ATM's or gasoline pumps. Shred as appropriate.

☐ Memorize passwords, PINS, and social security numbers. Do not record them or keep them in your wallet or purse.

☐ Sign all new credit cards upon receipt.

☐ Match credit card receipts with monthly bills.

☐ Be conscious of when financial statements are due and follow-up with the sender if they're late.

☐ Never loan your credit cards to anyone.

☐ Never put credit card or other financial account numbers on the outside of an envelope.

☐ If a new credit card does not arrive in a timely manner, call the issuer.

☐ Report lost or stolen credit cards immediately.

☐ Monitor expiration dates on credit cards. Contact the issuer if replacement cards are not received prior to expiration dates.

☐ Beware of solicitations offering an instant prize if you need to provide personal information, such as credit card numbers.

☐ Use caution when disclosing checking account numbers or credit card numbers with electronic services.

Credit Reports may be obtained from:

☐ Equifax, PO Box 105873, Atlanta, GA 30348-5873, Telephone: **1.800.997.2493**

☐ Experian Information Solutions, PO Box 949, Allen, TX 75013-0949, Telephone: **1.888.397.3742**

☐ TransUnion, PO Box 390, Springfield, PA 19064-0390, Telephone: **1.800.916.8800**

If You Are a Victim of Identity Theft

Some identity thieves can be successful even though you take necessary precautions. Insiders with companies sometimes provide thieves with information needed to commit fraud or theft. Take action immediately if you suspect your personal data has been stolen or misappropriated. According to the Federal Trade Commission, your first three steps should be:

1) Contact the Fraud departments of each of the three major credit bureaus. Advise them you are a victim of identity theft. Request that a "fraud alert" be placed in your file in addition to a victim's statement asking that creditors call you before opening any new

accounts or changing your existing accounts. Also, request copies of your Credit Report from each agency. Follow-up with a written request. Review your reports to make sure there are no additional fraudulent accounts.

2) Contact the creditors for any accounts that have been tampered with or opened fraudulently. Ask to speak with someone in the security or fraud department of each creditor, get their address, and follow-up with a letter. You must notify credit card companies in writing because the law requires you to do so in the consumer protection procedure for resolving errors on credit card billing statements. Immediately close accounts that have been tampered with, and open new accounts with new PIN's and passwords. Try to use a combination of numbers and letters, with seven characters or more for added protection.

3) File a report with your local police or the police in the community where the identity theft took place. Get a copy of the Police Incident Report or report number in the event the bank or credit card company needs verification that the police have been notified.

Other Steps to Take

If an identity thief has stolen your mail for fraud or theft, report it to the US Postal Service. Close all accounts the thief has tampered with and open new accounts, adding a password access for inquiries or changes to the accounts, banks, and investments included.

☐ The Federal Trade Commission (FTC) collects complaints about identity theft from consumers who have been victimized, and refers complaints to other appropriate government agencies and private organizations for further action.

☐ The FTC Identity Theft hotline is Toll Free **1.877.438.4338** or www.consumer.gov/idtheft. They also offer a number of valuable publications.

3 Federal Trade Commission, February 2002. " ID Theft – When Bad Things Happen to your Good Name"

4 US Postal Inspection Service – "Ensuring Confidence in the US Mail"

Section Six – General Safety Precautions

- CHAPTER 16 - WEAPONS FOR DEFENSE
- CHAPTER 17 - CARJACKING
- CHAPTER 18 - PERSONAL THREATS

Introduction

Everyone needs to be concerned about personal safety. But often people don't have the time or energy to worry about it as much as they should. Plus, no one wants to live life in fear or paranoia when they could be spending time with their family and friends, or doing things they love. But sometimes bad things happen without notice. Then when the unexpected occurs, the results can be devastating, especially to those who are completely unprepared.

However, awareness can reduce the risk of becoming a victim. So simply by increasing awareness of the existing vulnerabilities and potential areas a criminal may strike, people can better defend themselves and better recover from losses. The following chapters will help everyone increase their awareness and boost their defenses against unscrupulous predators.

Chapter 16
WEAPONS FOR DEFENSE

Self-defense should not depend on one strategy, such as running away, blowing a whistle to attract attention, or martial arts training. An effective strategy should consider that the primary action might not be completely effective in reaching the desired goal. Thus, a combination of defenses seems to be the optimal approach for everyday life.

Self Defense Classes - Practical Usefulness

A one-time women's self-defense class may be informative; however, practically speaking, it is of little value in the long run. Many of these types of classes are modified martial arts programs, which are complex and unrealistic under attack situations. To be an effective tool, techniques must be mastered and practiced on a fully-padded instructor in realistic attack scenarios. With regular follow-up practice, this defense tactic becomes a long-term commitment.

Chemical Spray

Pepper spray and mace, like other tools, may be useful as a defense against an attacker. However, unlike law enforcement officers who keep these agents readily available on their duty belt, most civilians do not have ready access to the canister. Additionally, these agents do not work on everyone to the same degree, may be affected by wind conditions, and direction of spray is not always accurate. However, pepper spray and mace can be effective tools provided they are readily available and conditions are good. Keep in mind that many jurisdictions have training requirements for chemical agents and laws regulating their use.

Hand Guns

Universally, laws regulate firearms of all types, and in particular, concealable handguns. These laws indicate the seriousness of carrying a handgun. Additionally, significant training, practice, and knowledge regarding appropriate use of a firearm are absolutely essential. Those considering a handgun as a defense method should also consider how they plan to keep it away from children when it isn't being carried. Ultimately, handguns are for deadly force. One must be willing to take a human life and also deal with the trauma that follows. And these are not small issues. If any of the above safety considerations are unacceptable, forget about carrying a handgun.

If you accept this responsibility, the next step is to enroll in a firearm's safety class. Here you should learn laws pertaining to use of deadly force, how to use the weapon, practice with the weapon, and maintenance of the weapon, among others. Additional supervised private instruction is also recommended.

You are not completely trained until you can keep all shots within the target zone while under stress. Stress is generally a timed, competitive situation. This training provides the knowledge and skill needed to qualify to carry a concealed handgun, but does not mean that it is recommended.

Chapter 17 CARJACKING

Carjacking is a completed or attempted theft of a motor vehicle by force or threat of force. It differs from other motor vehicle theft in that it only includes incidents in which the offender uses force or threats of force as defined by the US Department of Justice. Carjacking is a crime of opportunity — an opportunity to gain access to an item to exchange for quick cash, for drugs, or for use in another crime.

Several thousand completed or attempted carjackings occur each year. Many involve weapons and injury to occupants. They occur day and night in parking lots, at restaurants, office complexes, and other locations, and the majority happen relatively close to the victim's home.

High Risk Situations

As previously mentioned, a carjacking can occur anywhere, and at anytime. However, some situations increase risk. Generally any stopping event in traffic such as controlled intersections or stop signs increase vulnerability. Busy environments such as gas stations, car washes, and grocery stores offer cover for predators to attack with force or the threat of force and take the vehicle.

Another ruse is to get the driver to pull off the roadway by motioning or telling them something is wrong with their vehicle, or by slightly bumping the vehicle to get the driver to pull on to the shoulder. In either of the above, the thief's partner jumps into the victim's vehicle and both cars drive off.

Risk Reduction around Your Car

Plan ahead. Be aware. Previous chapters mentioned methods of establishing an aura or presence that may discourage the predator from choosing you as a victim. A few of these methods include: walk up right with a sense of purpose, have car keys at the ready position, look around, be cautious of vans, look inside your car before getting in, and don't become distracted.

Risk Reduction While Driving

Be aware. Check the rear view mirror often to detect if someone may be following you. Keep doors locked and windows rolled up high. Stay back from the car ahead of you on the road to leave an escape buffer, and don't stop for what may appear to be a disabled vehicle. If you do see a disabled car on the side of the road, drive out of the area and telephone police or use a cell phone to report the situation.

Risk Reduction When Parking

Park in well-lit areas, and anticipate darkness if your return to your vehicle will be after dark. Avoid parking near shrubbery or other potential concealment. Keep valuables in your car hidden out of view. Use attendant parking if possible.

Remember, seven out of ten carjackings involve firearms. If you come in contact with an armed carjacker, give them the car keys upon demand. Your life is more valuable than the vehicle.

Chapter 18

PERSONAL THREATS

A significant portion of private investigation is devoted to guiding people through the difficult events surrounding personal threats. These threats may be uttered in one-on-one conversations, anonymously by telephone, and sometimes by electronic mail. Threats are often vague in nature, but frequently are specific to some harmful action or actions. Regardless of the nature of the threat or the communication method, the recipient usually becomes very frightened and in almost all cases requests protection from the police and/or a private investigator.

From an intervention perspective, the immediate action by a private investigator is to assess the likelihood of imminent danger to the victim and his/her family, or others. This activity involves review and evaluation of the threat communication. The evaluation will define the nature and scope of protective and investigative measures to execute. These measures may include actions to:

- [ ] Facilitate law enforcement involvement;
- [ ] Facilitate acquisition of a restraining order;
- [ ] Recommend protective strategies for the threatened victim;
- [ ] Background the threat-maker, if possible;
- [ ] Obtain a psychological evaluation on the threat statement;
- [ ] Establish protective detail;
- [ ] Establish an incident team if the threat is work-related.

Law enforcement involvement is essential, providing the threat meets the threshold of a criminal violation. If a criminal violation exists, law enforcement will begin their process to make an arrest. During this period, protection may be required for the victim at work and at home. Upon arrest, the arrestee is most often subject to bail. If bail is posted, the person will be released; therefore, the protection agency must track these events and keep the victim informed on the status of the accused. Frequently, threats are made from the jail, or after release on bail. These should be brought to the attention of the law enforcement agency for additional action.

A Temporary Restraining Order (TRO) may be an appropriate remedy when one person threatens another. But the process for obtaining a TRO may vary slightly by geography. In California, the process begins with an application from a Superior Court. This application establishes which court has jurisdiction, who the plaintiff is, who the defendant is, and what the defendant has done. It requests that the court issue a TRO pending a future hearing. It also names the person or persons involved and specifically identifies the behaviors prohibited, such as:

☐ Must not threaten, strike, or make contact;

☐ Must not survey the victim;

☐ Must not block movements in public places;

☐ Must not follow;

☐ Must not telephone or send messages.

Additionally, stay-away orders require the defendant to stay some distance away (distance to be described) from:

☐ The plaintiff (the person threatened);

☐ The plaintiff's residence;

☐ The plaintiff's place of work;

☐ The plaintiff's children.

Declarations may be attached that support the defendant's actions or behavior. If the judge signs the TRO, a future court date is set for the defendant to give legal reasons why the orders sought should not be granted.

The TRO is civil in nature; however, a violation of this Order is criminal and therefore can be enforced by law enforcement officers. Restraining Orders should be viewed as an important part of a resolution in personal threat issues, however not the total answer. Because Restraining Orders are often ignored and subsequently violated, victims must not rely on them completely for protection. After all, the TRO is only a piece of paper and not a shield. As previously mentioned, the TRO is civil in nature and only after it is violated can the process move forward for a criminal violation and subsequently enforceable by the police.

TRO's are not gender specific. In August 2004, a woman in California was found guilty of stalking in violation of a court order, among other crimes dating back through years 2001 to 2003. She faces imprisonment for these violations.

Generally legal counsel is available to expedite Restraining Orders if necessary. Each of these resources provides valuable information and/or assistance from which an appropriate threat assessment can be made and in particular, to determine protective manpower requirements. Often multiple people and locations must be covered twenty-four hours a day, seven days a week.

Protective strategies for the threatened include many of the security suggestions offered in previous chapters. Additionally, protective strategies should be proportionate to threat evaluation or risk assessment. For example, if a threat is directed to a supervisor of a work group of several employees, then proportionate protection would be directed at the person who received the threat. Disproportionate protection would be to initiate 24/7 protection for the entire work group.

Awareness of your surroundings becomes even more important in threat situations. Vulnerable activity (i.e., going to and from work, shopping, and spending time in public places) must be reviewed and a mitigating scenario developed. If the threat is life threatening, mitigation could include an armed agent hired to protect your life and property. But if the threat is not life threatening, such as annoying phone calls, mitigation may be changing the phone number and not listing the number.

Criminal background checks may offer intelligence in regard to previous threat involvement or other violent crimes. For example, the background check could show a history of violence with a particular weapon. Obviously, this sort of information would be helpful in protection considerations because it provides insight into what the person is capable of doing.

In an employment situation, employers may require a "fit for work" evaluation (where permitted). This type of evaluation is designed to determine if the employee should be returned to the workplace in regard to his previous behavior. Psychological evaluations are also very valuable, and offer considerable insight into determining the credibility of a threat. Clearly, all threat events do not offer this possibility; however, if available, this information can be critical in developing a protective plan.

Personal Threats at Work

Business leaders and employers often use background checks to evaluate threats in the workplace. Aggressive behavior revealed through the background check may indicate a need to deploy a protective detail for employee layoffs or terminations. Other deployments may be non-business in nature, but in response to spouse/lover disputes of an employee that flows over to the workplace. In the former instance, a fair amount of intelligence gathered from the background check can evaluate a possible threat. Human Resource Department files often contain a pre-employment background screening report on the prospective employee. It, along with an employment application or resume, may indicate things such as military service. Additionally, it may include special military assignments such as Navy Seals or Special Forces. Obviously, this information could substantiate the skill requirement to carry out a physical threat.

In domestic issues, employers may become involved because an employee's intimate relationship has gone sour. Generally, these situations involve an errant love affair between an employee and a spouse, a boyfriend/girlfriend, or ex-lover that overflows into the workplace. Often threats of physical harm are made toward the employee, and the employer must take action to keep the workplace safe for all. These cases can be particularly troublesome for the employer. Besides the extra costs of safety measures, employers lose money in employee relations because of disruptions in focus and employees becoming concerned for their safety. Additionally, the employer has very little control over the situation in terms of resolution. To further complicate the issue for the employer, the issue often involves a romantic relationship between two employees and a non-employee. Many times while they are at work, the employees are often threatened harm by the non-employee.

Love is not always the instigator of these threats at work. A recent case involved a gambling situation that originated in the workplace. This particular work group was a tight-knit ethnic group, and the employer prohibited gambling in the workplace. Each week, the contributors gave a designated workgroup member money to place bets on their behalf at a casino in Lake Tahoe, Nevada. All went well for the workgroup until one member lost a large sum and borrowed money from a co-worker to conceal her gambling losses from her family. Her losses continued, and her debt became impossible to repay. The moneyman began to pressure the debtor, which impacted her work performance in addition to the workgroup's productivity.

Chapter 18 - Personal Threats

Then one evening as her spouse waited in the company parking lot to pick her up after work, he was accosted and beat up by two men of the same ethnicity as the workgroup. Ultimately, she quit her job to escape threats, but the employer lost a worker and suffered loss of productivity for a significant period of time.

Employers can avoid these situations by organizing Incident Teams. These Incident Teams are made up of multi-disciplinary professionals who deal with violence or threats of violence in the workplace. The central member is usually a psychologist or psychiatrist who is specifically trained to evaluate a potential risk. Other members may include a legal professional to ensure a worker's legal rights are not violated, a human resource professional to ensure a worker's company rights are not violated, a security professional to offer recommendations for protection of the threatened, and other employees.

Incident Teams may look different because of a company's size, structure, and procedures. Large companies may have resources such as security, human resources, legal, facilities, and medical personnel. But smaller companies may need consultation in these areas.

Incident Teams are responsible for dealing with any act or threat of violence in the workplace. Clearly, these incidents will have a range of potential. An immediate threat such as, "I'm going home to get my gun and come back and shoot that _ _ _ _," requires notification of law enforcement as soon as possible for intervention. But an Incident Team may be activated after law enforcement action for post evaluation and action.

In less serious events, the Incident Team is chartered to: evaluate the threat itself, its validity, its credibility, and to evaluate the person responsible for the threat. From these evaluations, an Incident Team develops information for senior managers to make informed decisions for moving forward.

For example, should the Incident Team conclude a valid credible threat exists and that the person may act out the threat, they may suggest increased physical security at the company and perhaps even personal security for the affected employee or employees. Another suggestion may be to offer the persons in danger security escorts to and from their vehicles while at work. These are examples of a few security suggestions the Incidents Team might develop. Other activities of the Incident Team could be:

- [ ] To develop press releases;
- [ ] To develop employee communications;
- [ ] To develop a termination letter for the threat-maker;
- [ ] To coordinate the event with law enforcement officials.

Think Safe

Many other considerations involved in dealing with threats, intimidation, or violence in the workplace exist. This information is intended to promote awareness in employers so they may recognize the advantages of pro-active planning in these issues.

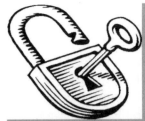

Section Seven – Crime Prevention

- CHAPTER 19 - PROTECTING THE HOME
- RESIDENTIAL SECURITY SURVEY

Introduction

Most police agencies, particularly in metropolitan areas, suffer from disparity between the number of uniformed personnel available and the number of calls requesting their service. Despite increased efficiency and technology, the demands for police service escalate each year in excess of the increases in manpower. These issues motivate police officials to seek other methods to serve and protect their communities, without additional personnel. Two strategies that address the demands for service while strengthening the police/community relationship are: community policing and crime prevention.

Community policing is structured slightly different in each community. However, the underlying principle is to get the officers who work a particular geographic area more in touch with people who live there, and vice versa. Through this close association between the police and community, the community is exposed to the problems of the police, and the police become aware of community issues concerning crime in their neighborhood. Together, this sharing of information promotes better reporting of the details police need to respond to crimes, and a better opportunity for the police to respond and apprehend criminals. It also allows the police to focus on chronic problems in the community, such as speeding, youth problems, or drug dealing.

The concept of crime prevention requires community involvement through vigilance for each other. The people in the community must report neighborhood crime, and to work toward removing opportunities for crime in their neighborhoods. Crime prevention also requires a partnership between law enforcement and the community. There simply aren't enough police officers to deal with all crime in all neighborhoods all of the time. Nor are communities equipped to substitute police officers to protect their communities. But by cooperating with each other, community members and police officers can help fight crime the most effective way, that is, before it begins.

Crime prevention targets opportunity. By removing opportunity, or significantly inhibiting opportunity, a crime is less likely to occur. An example could be the sexual predator that enters a home through open windows or unlocked patio doors on a warm summer night. If this intruder is met by a protective German shepherd, their desire and ability remain, but the dog takes away opportunity. In this situation, even though a break-in crime has been committed, it's not as serious as the intruder originally intended. The point is, by taking away opportunity for crime events, a safer environment is achieved.

Chapter 19   PROTECTING THE HOME

Burglary is among the most common major property crime reported to police. By its very nature, a crime of stealth, is not only difficult to prevent, but also difficult to clear by arrest. Phenomenal growth in population and land area further increase demands for municipal services, in addition to police service, to grow proportionately. If the crime of burglary is to be reduced, appropriate programs must be implemented by police agencies in partnership with the community.

This police-community partnership should set clearly identified goals and responsibilities for each. The police role and responsibility may include things like identifying areas of the city that experience high frequency crime, and high risk hours of the day and days of the week to assist in crime prevention efforts.

Another police activity may involve the development of performance metrics to determine effectiveness of specific activities designed to diminish a particular crime problem. For example, every burglar provides certain kinds of information that is useful in the fight against crime after entry and completion of a theft. The two principle uses of this information are: to prevent future thefts by knowing what items are commonly stolen, which makes possible implementation of specific programs to deter losses before they occur; and to identify conversion channels for recovering property after it has been stolen (and sometimes to identify the offender as well).

Further, knowing the frequency and items most commonly taken is valuable for establishing a base from which objective crime preventive measures can be established.

Past data shows that the majority of residential burglaries occur through forced entry. Thus, the primary objective of a burglary prevention project should be to do whatever possible (considering ability to pay) to focus on exterior things that make it more difficult for the burglar to gain entrance. Exterior things can be approached from objective and subjective methods. Objective methods are related to hardware such as case hardened padlocks, deadbolt locks, etc. Subjective methods are related more to the psychology of the thief, but are not totally divorced from hardware methods.

To illustrate, it is obvious that the most sophisticated security hardware device could be defeated by the cunning of a single person or persons with the proper equipment. Psychological deterrents can substantially strengthen any given level of physical deterrent. As an example of this effect, consider warning decals placed in selected areas advising the presence of an electronic burglar alarm. The fear of apprehension produced by such a warning will certainly influence the potential burglar whether or not there is an alarm present. This, of course, does not suggest that warning decals should be relied upon to protect property, only that a psychological barrier may act as a deterrent for the inexperienced, or sometimes experienced, thief.

The psychological contribution of the hardware used to prevent burglary is often overlooked, but is usually more important than the physical barrier it constructs. Lighting is a good example. The existence of lighting does not physically impair a burglar, but it certainly reduces the opportunity to steal, and also increases the fear of detection and arrest. From a burglar's viewpoint, a well-lit area is less attractive than a dark area. The psychological impact is lessened if an area is not well-lit and also offers dark parking places. Conversely, the impact is strengthened if a well-lit area is free of large shrubs that conceal activity, or if an alarm system is present.

In summary, burglary prevention efforts should provide a combination of hardware protection and psychological impact. The more coordinated the protection, the greater the awareness of reduced opportunity by the would-be offender, and the greater the psychological impact. Thus psychological impact is of particular significance and an essential consideration when discussing physical hardware security.

A burglar's forced entry is directly dependent on the types of locks, doors, and windows utilized by builders in home construction. Historically, cost consciousness has been the primary consideration in quality of materials used in homes, apartments, etc. In order to address this issue, consider two primary factors: construction methods must be modified, or home owners must reinforce with hardware those areas where the burglar is most likely to gain entrance.

Legislative action to establish construction building security codes is a lengthy, time-consuming process at best. Significant improvement has been made with building codes across the board; however doors, windows and locking devices continue to be weak points in home vulnerability. Thus, the most immediate answer seems to be employment of supplemental physical security measures. Physical security is generally described in terms of door and window systems, lighting, and electronic intrusion detection systems. The security function of each method is described in the accompanying table by the relationship between security measures and the security functions each perform. These functions cover the principal necessities of residential security, short of force by residents to protect themselves.

The Relationship between Physical Security Measures and Security Functions

Physical Security Measures (Hardware)	Access Control	Control of Forced Entry	Control of Other Crime	Reduction Of Escape Possibilities	Psychological Deterrence
Door and Window Systems	x	x	x	x	x
Intrusion Detection Systems		x	x	x	x
Exterior Lighting	x	x	x	x	x

The functions are designed to highlight security objectives and are arranged in an order by which a burglar could evaluate a target.

The degree to which any hardware security device attains the intended objective is the degree to which a home becomes "unattractive" as a burglary target. Therefore, the utility of a security device should be considered not only by its intrinsic value, but also by the effect it will produce on other security measures with which it is used.

Security Devices and Systems

A myriad of security devices and systems are used for commercial and residential purposes, and these become the subject of many crime articles, books, and crime prevention informative literature throughout the country. The following list describes the most common security hardware for residential security:

1. Doors

Many factors contribute to the vulnerability of a door besides the lock that secures it. Whether the door is made of wood or metal, solid or hollow-core, how well it fits into the frame, and many other factors determine how resistant a door is to forced entry. And many different kinds of doors are utilized in residential use. The types of doors and the materials used vary from neighborhood to neighborhood, from area to area, and from builder to builder.

Because of these variables, and also the quality of craftsmanship used in manufacturing processes, describing a door that provides optimal security for all residences or for all kinds of security needs is not practical. The vulnerability of a door is usually thought of in terms of it penetrability, and is akin to the burglary resistance rating assigned to safe vaults. That is, how long would it take a person to penetrate the door, when supplied with all the necessary tools.

The ability to penetrate, however, is not a significant factor in illegal entry. In fact, breaking through a door is not the most common method employed for defeating a door system. Loose doors in the frame are a much more significant factor because the improper fit allows the door to be pried or forced open with greater ease.

Builders use several types of doors for the primary entrance. Of these, the four major types include:

☐ Flush wood doors;

☐ Fiberglass;

☐ Half (or partial) glass and wood doors;

☐ Metal doors.

Flush wood doors can also be broken into two types: hollow-core and solid core. A hollow-core door is nothing more than two sheets of a very thin material, usually plywood with overlapping cardboard strips. Despite the obvious ease of penetrating a hollow-core door, they are used in abundance as exterior doors because they are less expensive than other more-durable types.

On the other hand, solid-core doors offer a considerable security advantage over hollow-core doors. The name, solid-core, describes the interior components of this type of door. Generally, these components are particles of wood glued together to form a solid mass. Solid-core doors are often used between the house and garage for protection from fire, as well as for security. Fiberglass doors are similar to solid-core doors.

Half or partial glass doors also come in a variety of shapes and forms. The obvious weakness in these exterior doors is the presence of glass. Simply by breaking the glass, the intruder can reach in and unlock the deadbolt, or other security device in use. Also, this type of door must fit snug in its frame to defeat a prying or forcing action.

From a security standpoint, a steel-sheathed door is superior to any and all types of wood door. A steel door is usually mounted on a steel frame reinforced with interior braces. The main objection to metal doors is usually aesthetic, as they are generally less attractive than wood doors. However, because of the superior strength of steel over wood, metal doors are usually recommended when they can be worked into the architectural design, without becoming a significant cost factor.

2. Windows and Sliding Glass Doors

Windows and sliding glass doors cause a host of security problems. Windows and sliding glass doors come in a great variety of styles and sizes, and are designed for appearance rather than security. The type or style of window is largely predicated on the ventilation or light/heat it affords, with less consideration for security objectives. And for the most part, only when a well-placed window makes vulnerable areas observable does it add any security value.

In all other respects, windows decrease security. This, of course, varies in degrees because some windows are more vulnerable than others. Variables such as size of the panes, distance from ground level, and fixed or hinged openings are significant factors. The one common factor is all windows are breakable, unless they are made of burglar-resistant glass.

The vulnerability of window areas tends to be inversely related to the vulnerability of main entry doors. Almost any intruder will try to get through the doors before resorting to windows. Little data is available on the odds of a burglar breaking glass to gain entrance. But most burglars are apprehensive about the noise made by shattering glass, and they are concerned about injuring themselves in the process of gaining entry through broken windows.

In many windows and glass doors, the locking mechanism can be successfully manipulated from the outside. Techniques, such as inserting an object between the window and sill, are sufficient to release the locking device. Once this is accomplished, forcing the window open without breaking the glass becomes easy.

Louvered windows tend to be particularly vulnerable; no practical way to prevent them from being pried open to gain access to a door handle exists. Two methods are generally employed to protect vulnerable windows: First, steel bars or grillwork outside the windows; and second, installation of tempered glass in the louvered panes. However, neither method offers optimum satisfaction.

Although attractive, steel bars or grillwork block the transmission of light, thus interfering with one of the basic purposes of the window. Tempered glass is often considered because of its resistance to shattering, but the security value is relatively low. Tempered glass will resist a brick or a rock, but is vulnerable to sharp objects. And when attacked, tempered glass tends to crumble away quietly, rather than shatter loudly, which eliminates some element of danger to the intruder.

3. Lighting

A basic approach to reducing nighttime crime is the introduction of light into the area. This can be as simple as placing a porch light over the back door to a residence, or as complicated as illuminating a baseball field for evening television coverage. But outdoor lighting can be one of the most effective deterrents against crime. Properly used, lighting can discourage criminal attacks, increase observer ability, and dramatically reduce fear and apprehension in a community.

Universal lighting standards that would be widely applicable to residential neighborhoods are difficult to conceive. In many neighborhoods, streetlights cast enough light to provide reasonable observation ability between the roadway and front entryways. But foliage, fences, and other man-made barriers often impair the adequacy of street lighting. When these items are present and street lighting does not provide sufficient illumination, porch lights and other exterior lighting supplied by the home owner will usually suffice. Additional lights can be placed over garages and driveways to provide adequate observation ability from inside the house, and for walking from the street or garage into the house. As a general rule, the amount of light needed for security will allow a person to perceive a threat from any direction.

On the other hand, one of the greatest risks to home safety is improper or excessive lighting: a too well-lit area can be dangerous because of the inability to see beyond the illuminated area. Thus, the most critical problem in residential neighborhoods is not the level of brightness, but rather the evenness of light. To prevent such instances of uneven lighting, supplemental light sources of a lesser intensity should be deployed around the perimeter to assist in eye adjustment. Under most circumstances, lighting patterns should be designed to provide smooth transitions between well-lit, marginally-lit, and dark areas.

It seems reasonable to conclude that lighting has a profound influence on crime reduction. Similar conclusions can be drawn on the effect of lighting and the potential burglar. But to discuss the effects of lighting on the crime of burglary, a short review of the known methods of operation, or known characteristics of burglars are appropriate.

By its very definition, burglary is a crime against property. Thus, it follows that confrontation by the burglar with homeowners or apartment dwellers is not likely. As a matter of fact, in most cases the burglar will go to considerable lengths to make sure that the residence they intend to burglarize is unoccupied at the time of the break-in. This is carried out in several ways, one of which is phoning the prospective residence at a certain time of day for a specific time period. If no one answers each time a call is placed, the burglar will choose that time and day in a subsequent week to commit the crime. Burglars even pose as salesmen, repairmen, charity solicitors, and servicemen – all to the end of ensuring a vacant dwelling.

Lights at night act, at the very least as illumination of prospective targets. For either the burglar that will strike as the opportunity presents itself, or the burglar that extensively plans his attack, lights provide indices from which to gage occupancy. The likelihood that a well-lit home is occupied is far greater than a home that is dark. Thus, the presence or absence of light could be the first factor the burglar considers when choosing a target.

Perimeter and Structural Security

The elements discussed thus far, doors, doorframes, windows, and lighting, form the basic and minimal ingredients of a residential security system. That is, doorframes should be inspected and tested, window casements may be checked for weakness, and effective lighting systems can be installed or improved. These components make up a significant portion of the security environment that exists in a residential area.

For the purpose of definition, a security environment means the minimal security system that should be incorporated into all the homes of a residential community that will produce reasonable expectations of protection from burglars of opportunity, first time offenders, etc. Minimum security means the prevention of entry by a burglar through any door or window, except by use of destructive force.

These elements could broadly be categorized as perimeter and structural security. Perimeter environmental elements include such things as shrubbery trimmed away from windows, mail and newspapers collected on a regular basis, and exterior lighting in the front and rear of the residence.

Structural security elements include extra measures, such as deadbolt locks installed on all doors front and back, patio sliding glass door locks, windows protected by supplemental locks, light timers in use when home is unoccupied, key security, door viewer, and perhaps an alarm system. These elements are hardware items and are available to consumers in a variety of configurations.

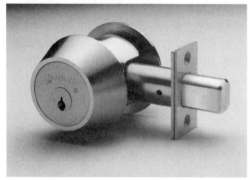

Deadbolt locks such as the one picture left have four critical parts: the housing, the internal mechanism, the bolt length, and the tumbler system. Unfortunately, the greater number of security features a deadbolt lock has, the greater the cost. Cost is generally a consideration for homeowners, and in some cases, the only consideration. However, cost will be disregarded from this section, as the security afforded by the locking device is the issue.

The housing of the deadbolt lock should be of solid construction to act as a rigid barrier, and case hardened steel is recommended. The cylinder should be assembled using one-quarter inch case hardened steel bolts. It should be designed in a curved contour that wards off clamping tools, or have a cylinder guard that rotates with any attempt to twist the lock off. No screw heads should exist on the exterior face, and the bolt throw should be at least one inch in length.

The tumbler system of a lock refers to the tiny metal pins of varying lengths that determine the combination of the cylinder. The more pin tumblers in a lock increase the degree of difficulty in picking it. Generally, a five-pin tumbler is adequate for residential security.

In simple terms, double cylinder means a key on both sides. These locks are commonly used in doors that have a window within forty inches of the locking device because they prevent a person from breaking the glass and extending their arm or other instrument inside to unlock the door. A downside to this lock is escape during an emergency may be impossible without a key.

A single cylinder deadbolt lock is very similar to the double cylinder except a throw replaces one of the key sides. Either of these locks should have a one-inch bolt length. Finally, a dead latch locking device does little more than protect against a plastic card from slipping the door open.

Double doors present a particular problem because of the way they open, and the inherent weakness where the doors meet at the center. In order to properly secure these kinds of doors, the inactive side must be reinforced. Generally, contractors use half-barrel slide-bolts on the inactive door. However, these are weak and inadequate. A cane bolt, one-half inch in diameter by twelve inches high, should be installed at the top and bottom of the inactive door to offer minimum security. Flush bolts installed at the top and bottom of the inactive door provide additional security over cane bolts, since the intruder cannot access these devices to tamper with them if the doors are locked.

Another locking device as equally effective and less expensive than a deadbolt is the rim lock. The rim lock is a one-inch deadbolt lock which is installed on the inside surface of the door. It also comes available in a "jimmy-proof" model that has vertical deadbolts to provide additional security.

One last area of concern for the protection of the double door is the hinge position. First of all, if practical, the hinge should face inside the home, because any knowledgeable intruder can remove many so-called non-removable hinge pins fairly easily. Once the hinge pins are removed, the intruder simply lifts the door out of place.

If the hinges face outward, simple steps can be taken to protect the door from being lifted from its hinges. First, remove the two screws, opposite each other, from both leaves of the hinge. Next, insert a screw or concrete nail into jamb (post) leaf so it protrudes half an inch. Then, drill out the opposing screw hole in the door. Repeat this in the top and bottom hinges of the door. Then when closed, the pins may be removed, but the door will remain firmly in place. This technique, along with a double cylinder lock can also convert an almost useless small bedroom closet into a secure cabinet for storage of items away from children.

The purpose of securing a sliding glass door is to prevent the door from being pried up and out of the track. Wooden rods or metal bars may be placed in the track to prevent the door from opening, but a burglar could remove these using specially formed wires inserted beneath the door track. Also, once the intruder has gained entrance to the premises from another door or window, he can easily remove these rods or bars and use this exit to remove large items.

Consideration of fire danger and exit ways for an occupied home should always take priority over locked doors and windows. But in an unoccupied home, you don't have to worry about escaping emergencies and security can become your primary concern. Following are suggestions for an unoccupied home. A simple way to secure an inside sliding door is to drill a downward sloping hole through the top channel into the top portion of the sliding door frame and insert a pin. This method may be used when the home is unoccupied, but when the home is occupied, a door that doesn't open becomes too big a risk.

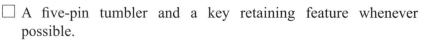

Another way to secure a sliding door is to install a slide bolt. To offer additional security when the home is unoccupied, a padlock keyed to the front door may be added. Many other devices are available for securing sliding doors. However, those referred to above offer an inexpensive, effective security measure.

Attached garages also provide an easy method of entry for intruders. This poses a particular problem because most garages have an entry into the residence from the garage. In addition, many homeowners keep a supply of tools stored in the garage that an intruder may use to attack other locking mechanisms. Many garages are secured by only one lock, which often permits an intruder to pry up the opposite side of the door and crawl under.

Methods to secure a garage are:

1) Add another bolt and padlock to the opposite side;

2) Install a pair of cane bolts to the inside;

3) Add a hasp at the top center of the door.

This hasp must be hardened steel and installed with carriage bolts through the door. Use large washers on the inside, and after the nuts are tightened, deface the bolt ends to prevent nut removal. And then add the padlock.

Many types and varieties of padlocks exist on the market. Economy, while a consideration, should have minimum weight in the selection process. The most common assault on a padlock is with a large bolt cutter or pry bar, thus the following are minimum requirements:

☐ The padlock should have a minimum 9/32 inch shackle of hardened steel;

☐ A double-locking mechanism – heel and toe;

☐ A five-pin tumbler and a key retaining feature whenever possible.

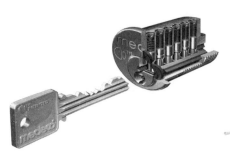

The five-pin tumbler (as pictured on left) feature prevents removal of the key until after the padlock has been locked. A padlock should never be left unlocked. An unlocked padlock is an invitation for the padlock to be removed and a key made. Also, padlock numbers should be recorded, and then defaced to prevent key duplication.

Window security is very similar to sliding glass door procedures. With sliding windows, the primary objective is to keep the window from sliding or being lifted out of the track. Many manufactured products are available for security windows, two of which are the anti-slide block and the slide bolt.

Avoid locking a window in a ventilating position, as this provides an opportunity to pry the window up and out. Contrary to sliding glass doors, key-locking devices offer no real security and they can become a fire exit hazard.

Casement windows, those that crank out, may be the simplest kind of window to secure. Just make sure the latch works properly and that the opening mechanism has no excess play. If either is not operable, they should be replaced.

Double hung window latches may be jimmied open, but at least two procedures will prevent this from happening. If the window is not used, and it is not a bedroom window, consider using several large wood screws to secure it permanently. For a window in use, drill a downward sloping hole into the top of the bottom window – through and into the bottom of the top window – and insert a pin or nail will secure the window. But remember fire danger, and never secure an exit that may be needed in case of an emergency.

Louvered windows are high security risks. If possible, they should be replaced with solid glass. When discussing window security, always remember that they are important escape routes in emergencies. At night, a bedroom window may be the quickest, safest, and only method of exit.

Underwriters Laboratory (UL®) and the American National Standards Institute (ANSI) establish protocols that locking devices (among many other items) must meet to achieve a rating from the organization. Other standards are set by law such as in the Americans with Disabilities Act (ADA). All standards are important, but for different reasons. UL® and ANSI standards assess usage, while ADA standards assess accessibility.

The security of any locking device depends on two critical factors:

☐ Physical strength against picking, drilling, and other forms of attack;

☐ Controlling keys and/or duplication of keys.

Unauthorized key duplication plays a major role in compromising even the most sophisticated security systems. Effective key control is essential to the success of a security lock system, and unfortunately most keys are easily duplicated. The warning "do not duplicate" stamped on a key only serves as a challenge for most non-professional key duplicators. If you can have keys copied at a local store, then a burglar can have your keys copied also. Clearly think through your lock requirements and select one that provides the level of protection and control that is appropriate to your needs.

Medeco, a maker of high security locks, provides many different levels of patented key protection:

☐ **Standard Commercial** offers physical protection available by the type of cylinder, but may not have patent-protected keys, and therefore no authorization to obtain duplicate keys is required.

☐ **Card Restricted** offers physical protection and utility patent-protected keys. Requires authorization card and signature verification to obtain duplicate keys, which are cut at a limited number of contract-controlled factory authorized service centers.

☐ **Contract Restricted** offers physical protection and utility patent- protected keys. A contract between the service outlet and the institution ensures strict adherence to key control policies, which require signature verification to obtain duplicate keys.

☐ **Factory Restricted** offers physical protection and utility patent-protected keys. All keys are cut at the factory with appropriate signature verification, and blanks are not released outside the Medeco factory.

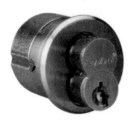

High security cylinders in Medeco's Biaxial® locks have earned a UL® listing, because they provide pick and drill resistance and utility patented key control. The Biaxial® lock design combines several unique features to create a high security lock that is virtually pickproof. Medeco Biaxial® locks provide exceptional security against physical attack.

Home Security – A Dog

An important consideration for home security is a dog. Small or large, dogs can play an important role in one's life as a pet and protector. The size and breed of dog is an issue of personal preference. In choosing a breed that suits your needs, make sure you consider your lifestyle and the amount of space you have for the dog to roam and play.

Dogs are an excellent property and personal protector. A bark can be enough to convince a potential burglar to keep moving, which may allow you more freedom and reduce apprehension about being away from home. In summary, a dog may be the best security available.

Another consideration is the detection value of the dog. A dog has an incredible sense of smell and hearing, which allows him to detect an intruder long before a human can, and in many circumstances before an alarm. Dogs are also nocturnal animals. This intrinsic nighttime awareness makes the dog an excellent protector during sleep. Most would agree that the dog is the most valuable protector of their human masters. Absent the ability to reason, a dog can put himself in harms way.

If you are considering specialty training for the dog, such as protective training, be aware of several factors. One, consider liability if the dog attacks someone inappropriately, or even in some cases appropriately. Two, some insurance companies cover one bite by the dog, but void subsequent coverage. Three, protective-trained dogs are expensive and require regular practice. Four, periodic training and handling are required to maintain necessary skills. Thus, except in a few special circumstances, the need for a protective-trained dog is nonexistent. Obedience training is preferable.

While dogs can effectively deter crime, any dog can become a nuisance or menace to a community. Careful thought should be given to the needs of the animal before purchase. If doubts about the compatibility of the animal to the household or community exist, consultation with a veterinarian can be helpful in understanding the basic needs of the animal. Additionally, a veterinarian can offer insight into time requirements for care, play, and training.

Property Identification

Despite precautions, loss of property to the crime of burglary is always a clear possibility. Thus, potential victims must be able to appropriately identify their belongings for at least three reasons:

- [ ] Police will need descriptions to attempt recovery;

- [ ] Insurance companies often require descriptions for claim purpose;

- [ ] To substantiate a claim for the property if recovered by a policy agency.

Two methods for property identification are by recording serial numbers and photography. Serial number recordation works very well for major electrical appliances, firearms, etc. Other items such as antiques, rings, and jewelry are excellent items to photograph. Also, the nature of these items often makes it very difficult for the owner to describe them for the police investigation. Additionally, photographing the entire content of the home is a good idea in case of a natural disaster in order to support claims.

If possible, use a digital camera and subsequently move the photos to a compact disc. Two copies, one kept at home and another away, such as a safety deposit box, works very effectively. In any event, photographs are easy to store in a safe or perhaps in an insurance folder at a broker's office. This also permits almost immediate retrieval.

Photographs accompanied by prompt reporting of loss to a policy agency also show validity of ownership. Many times proof of ownership poses a difficult issue when police recover property. In many states, by law, the person claiming recovered property must be able to clearly identify and prove ownership of it. If they are unable to do so, the police agency will not release the item(s) to the claimant.

Some other special advantages of photographic identification are earlier apprehension of a burglar, testimony in court, and expediting the law enforcement process.

Burglar Alarms

An alarm system offers several advantages – it may deter a crime, it may interrupt a crime, and it may detect a fire or intrusion and immediately report the event to authorities. But some disadvantages exist that must be incorporated into your decision to purchase an alarm system. In some communities, police and fire departments no longer respond to residential alarms because of a high frequency of false alarms. Alarms annoy neighbors, and children often forget about disengaging it and thus cause activation. If these disadvantages are not considered and resolved, when purchased, the alarm system will become valueless.

The installation of an alarm system must be approached with the same caution exercised with any major purchase. Check with other alarm owners, and avoid do-it-yourself installations. Also know the vendor, and consider how long they've been in the business. Finally, consider the security unit itself. Are replacement parts available? How often does it need to be serviced? Is back-up power on the system and system monitor available? Is it Underwriters Laboratory (UL) listed?

Many police agencies offer advice on alarm systems to the public. Also, contact your insurance carrier for advice and perhaps a reduction on insurance premiums.

Security Survey

In previous chapters, systems, methods, and techniques for an efficient home and personal protection/prevention program were discussed. Areas included locks, doors, lighting, property identification, security systems, and devices, etc. In order to evaluate a particular home on how it meets or doesn't meet minimum security recommendations, an inspection form proves very valuable While the inspection form and its contents may vary, the items to be considered and checked generally fall into perimeter and structural checkpoints. Perimeter considerations are items like shrubbery, exterior lighting, outside locks, door viewers, window protection,etc. Structural considerations are items such as locks, windows, doors, etc.

The purpose of the survey is to point out the vulnerability of a dwelling, to recognize and appraise the crime risk, and to incorporate recommendations to reduce or remove that vulnerability or crime risk. However, no matter how well-defined the purposes of a survey are, the ultimate benefit can only be realized if action is taken on the survey findings and conclusions. Clearly, the survey has the greatest value when conducted by a security professional; however, it is also of value to homeowners, realtors, and others as a starting point to focus on security deficiency. See the illustration in the appendix.

This sample survey form represents a starting point that can be expanded to cover other topics previously discussed throughout this book. A security professional would probably approach an inspection by establishing guidelines.

The first guideline for the surveyor should be to recognize the objectives of the survey and establish goals from which to work. As an example, one goal may be to create realistic expectations for the recipient on what can be accomplished with a security survey. Others may include establishing channels of communication involving all those affected by security risks; developing and communicating crime demographics of the community; establishing a plan of action; and motivating everyone involved to reduce the crime risk.

These goals are not necessarily in chronological order, and attainment of one might be dependent on attainment of another. Nevertheless, successful implementation of the survey depends largely on attaining positive results in these areas. After implementation, a periodic review should be made to account for changes in crime and crime patterns, family, neighbors, and other variables.

Think Safe

Residential Security Survey - Circle your answers

Around the Home

1) Is your home address visible from the street?   **Yes**   **No**
Goal: Address numbers are important for emergency vehicle response.

2) Are your shrubs and bushes trimmed around your home? **Yes**   **No**
Goal: Prevent easy concealment spaces for intruders by trimming all shrub from the ground up 3 to 4 feet.

3) Do you have proper lighting around the outside perimeter of your home?
Yes   **No**
Goal: Proper lighting discourages thieves and provides visibility at night.

4) Are your garage doors properly secured? **Yes**   **No**
Fact: Did you know that garage doors can be forced open, if they have inferior locking devices? Once an intruder gains access to a garage, they are then able to utilize your tools to break into the home.

5) Have you recently inspected the locks on other outside structures such as sheds and outdoor storage closets?
Yes   **No**
Fact: Vulnerability of outside storage areas my entice thieves to attack other personal property and structures.

6) While on vacation are your newspapers and mail collected? **Yes**   **No**
Fact: Presence of mail may indicate absence. Additionally mail left unattended or uncollected provides an opportunity for identity theft.

7) Do you have a home alarm system? **Yes**   **No**
Fact: Barking dogs can also be valuable for deterrence.

Doors

8) Are your doors well maintained? **Yes**   **No**
Consider the following:
Construction - Entry doors should be solid-core construction
Hinges - Non-removable pins facing inward
Locks - Case-hardened entry with at least 1" deadbolt with thumb turn inside.
Must be aware of fire safety

162

9) Are there door viewers installed on entry doors?
Yes   No
Important: Safety feature to use before opening doors.

10) Do you use light timers?
Yes   No
Goal: Gives the appearance of someone being home.

Windows

11) Are your windows well maintained?
Idea: Check the construction of your windows like you did your doors.

12) Are your windows protected by locks or grills?
Yes   No
Safety Warning: Grills or wrought iron bars are not generally recommended due to fire safety.

Securing Valuables

13) When having your car repaired do you hand over all your keys?
Yes   No
Comment: The correct answer here is NO. Do not include your house key with the car key. If you loss your house keys, re-key locks.

14) Do you engrave or mark personal items such as televisions and tools?
Yes   No
Idea: Items that cannot be etched/engraved with personal items such as diamonds, watches, etc., take photos and keep one set of photos outside the home.

CONCLUSION

Personal safety is a broad subject that everyone needs to be aware of, but it is also an ever-changing subject. As you move through your life and your situations change, your personal safety needs will change as well. This book encompasses a huge range of possibilities and preventions, but you don't have to be paranoid or afraid to live your life. Safety and security don't have to control your every single thought. But by becoming aware of what scams and dangers exist, and of the ways to protect yourself and what's important to you, you will make better decisions. And making better, more informed decisions is truly the foundation of personal security. When you use the information covered in this book to make better decisions you increase the safety and security in your own life, and in the lives of the people you love. You can be safe in all aspects of your life, but you must *think safe*.

Index

A

abductor 25–28
abusive xvii, 59, 75–78, 87, 101, 111
access 26, 29, 31, 39, 53, 54, 105–
     110, 124–137, 152, 155
alarm systems 161
alcohol 46, 62, 68, 86–87, 97, 98, 111
Americans with Disabilities Act 157
American Academy of Child & Ado-
     lescent Psychiatry 48
American National Standards 157
America Online 53
announcements 25–27
awareness 37, 43, 45, 59, 68, 73, 93,
     107, 119, 130, 133, 144, 148,
     159

B

babysitters 18, 50
background 29–34, 101, 110, 141, 142
badges 26
Bank Examiner Fraud 90
Better Business Bureau 125, 127
body language 63
Breaux, Senator 83–86
Bureau of Justice Statistics 42, 59, 63
burglary 94, 147–153, 159

C

Canadian Sweepstakes Scam 93
caregiver 32, 84, 87, 97, 98
carjacking 133–168
CDC 40
charities 125
child protection 39
Child Protection Act 29
Columbine School shooting 40
Comprehensive School Safety Act 37.
     known as HR 1216
courtesy victim 102
crime prevention 38, 44, 45, 69,

     145–147, 150
criminal xvii, 39, 61, 85, 91, 93, 110,
     133
criminologists xvii
Cybersitter 2000 54
Cybersnoop 54

D

date rape 62
   drugs 62
date rape, prevention 62, 68
Davis, Gray Governor 30
deadbolt locks 148, 154
Department of Education 44
Direct Marketing Association 128
disease 72
distraction burglary 94
domestic fraud 94
domestic violence 75–79
domestic violence, cycle of 79
do not call list 95
drink safe, technology 62, 63
Drug-Free Schools 44
dumpster diving 129

E

elder abuse 83–88
   preventing 86
emergency phone numbers 27
empower 59
Equifax 128, 131
evacuation plans 33
Experian 128, 131
exterior lighting 49, 152–168

F

Federal Trade Commission 122, 123,
     131, 132
Fingerprint 27
fingerprints 29
fire 59, 151, 155–158, 160
firearm. *See also* weapon
fire extinguishers 27
fire safety 94

fraud 84–88, 94–168
fraud prevention strategies 103

H

handgun 136. *See also* firearm, weapon
harassment 84, 115–117
healthcare 26
home repair 91
home security 27, 158
Home Security Checklist 69
home security survey 69
HR 1216 37
HR 1812 37

I

identification 70, 159–160
identification records 29
identity theft 129–132
illness 33, 48
incident team 139, 143
infant 25–28
injury 31, 34, 40, 92
Internet Fraud 99
intervention 34, 37, 46, 48
investment fraud 98
isolation 75, 79, 84–85, 97

L

law enforcement 42, 46, 65, 77, 79, 88, 100, 135, 139
light timer 27
locks 27–28, 49, 69, 148–152, 158–162

M

magazine subscriptions 95–97
medications 50
murder xvii, 19

N

National Center for Juvenile Justice 23
National Domestic Violence Hotline 79

National Incident-Based Reporting System 20
negotiation 45
Net Nanny 54
Nigerian Letter 127

O

Ohio State University Extension Fact Sheet 47–48

P

P.C. Magazine 54
paranoid 164
password 132
pepper spray 67, 72, 135
Pigeon Drop 90
Power of Attorney 89
predator 59–69, 89, 126, 138, 146
preventing elder abuse 87. *See also* elder abuse
prey vii, 81, 89–94, 102, 127
prosecution 73, 85
pyramid scheme 101

Q

quid pro quo sexual harassment 115

R

rape xvii, 19, 23, 30, 62. *See also* date rape
reporting investment fraud 103

S

safe house 39
San Jose Mercury News 68
School Anti-Violence Empowerment Act 37. *known as* HR 1812
Securities Exchange Commission 99, 101
sexual harassment 115, 116
sexual harassment, defination of 115
sexual harassment, hostile enviroment 115
sexual harassment complaint 115
sexual victimization 63
smoke detectors 27
Snyder, Howard PH.D. 23

sodomy 20, 21
stalker 62
Stefan, Ken 74
suicide intervention 46
Surf Control White Paper 54

T

Taylor, Christine 45, 46
telemarketing fraud 97
temporary restraining order 138
theft 87
Trans Union 126

U

Underwriters Laboratory 158
USA Today 38
US Department of Education 38

V

victimization 20, 37
victimization of children 38
victimization of seniors 87
victimization of teachers 39
violence, cycle of 74

W

weapon 70. *See also* firearm, handgun
weapons 44, 70, 135
Web Safety Tips 53

What You Need to Know to Live a Safe, Secure Life

"Jim's experience in law enforcement and security makes *Think Safe* a valuable and practical guide to personal and workplace safety and security."

— Broadus Durant (retired)
Hospital Security and Transportation Manager

Check with your neighborhood and online bookstores or order here.

Toll-Free: 1-866-372-2636

Secure Online Ordering www.CameoPublications.com

	# Items	Amount
Think Safe Paperback 168pp *(ISBN 0-9744149-6-4):* **$19.95**		
Shipping USA: $4.95 for first item;add $2.00 for each additional book/CD Canada: $6.00 for first item; add $4.00 for each additional book/CD SC residents please include 5% Sales Tax		
	Order Total	

Please Print

Name _____
Company _____
Ship To _____
City/State/Zip_____ Country _____

Phone ( ) _____ E-mail (optional) _____

MasterCard VISA AMERICAN EXPRESS DISCOVER

Cameo Publications
PO BOX 8006
Hilton Head, SC 29938

credit card # _____ expires _____

please sign _____